IF TODAY
Is
All I HAVE

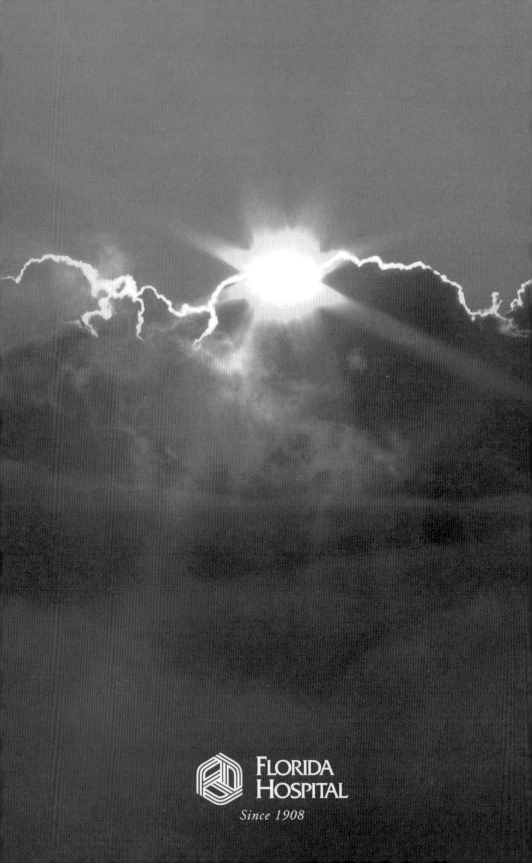

IF TODAY Is All I HAVE

*Finding the Light of Hope
in Dark Places*

LINDA NORDYKE HAMBLETON
with TODD HILLARD

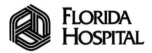

IF TODAY IS ALL I HAVE

TO EXTEND *the* HEALTH *and* HEALING MINISTRY *of* CHRIST

EDITOR-IN-CHIEF	Todd Chobotar
MANAGING EDITOR	David Biebel, DMin
BUSINESS DEVELOPMENT	Stephanie Lind, MBA
PROMOTION	Laurel Dominesey
PRODUCTION	Lillian Boyd
COPY EDITOR	Barbara Trombitas
COVER DESIGN	Tri Widyatmaka
INTERIOR DESIGN	Judy Johnson
PHOTOGRAPHER	Spencer Freeman

PUBLISHER'S NOTE: This book is not intended to replace a one-on-one relationship with a qualified health care professional, but as a sharing of knowledge and information from the research and experience of the author. You are advised and encouraged to consult with your health care professional in all matters relating to your health and the health of your family. The publisher and author disclaim any liability arising directly or indirectly from the use of this book.

AUTHOR'S NOTE: This book contains many patient stories and medical histories. In order to preserve the privacy of some of the people involved, I have disguised their names, appearances, and aspects of their stories so they are not identifiable. Patient stories may include composite characters.

For volume discounts please contact special sales at:
HealthProducts@FLHosp.org | 407-303-1929

*Cataloging-in-Publication Data for this book
is available from the Library of Congress.
Printed in the United States of America.*

PR 14 13 12 11 10 9 8 7 6 5 4 3 2 1
ISBN-13: 978-0-9839881-0-6

For more Whole Person Health resources visit:
**FloridaHospitalPublishing.com
Healthy100Churches.org
CreationHealth.com
Healthy100.org**

CONTENTS

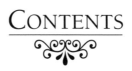

ABOUT THE AUTHOR

*L*INDA NORDYKE HAMBLETON was diagnosed with juvenile-onset diabetes (type I diabetes mellitus) at the age of six. Doctors gave her to age twenty-five to live. With dreams, pain, laughter, and tears, she exceeded their prediction by more than twenty years. Truly a model of physical, mental, and spiritual human survival, Linda writes from the heart with honesty and experience. It is a message of hope to all individuals and their loved ones who suffer from the chronic condition called "life."

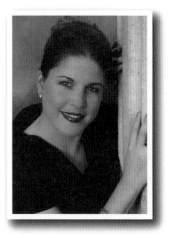

ABOUT THE COLLABORATOR

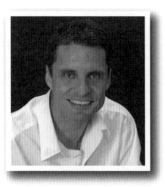

*T*ODD A. HILLARD is a freelance writer from San Antonio, Texas. The husband of one and the father of five, he spends his "spare" time making the thoughts and dreams of others come alive on the written page.

todd.hillard@gmail.com

FOREWORD

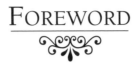

*L*INDA HAMBLETON WAS a woman of great faith. She set a marker for those of us who have suffered. In spite of unbelievable physical odds, Linda confidently said, "My heart is weak but full of gratitude." And she lived that. Her suffering was a testament to the presence and grace of the Lord Jesus.

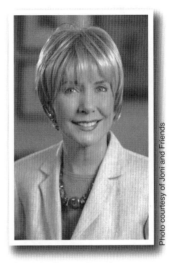

One of her anchors was the truth found in God's Word that I have embraced for so many years. "Be strong and courageous. Do not be afraid or terrified [of quadriplegia or diabetes], for the LORD your God goes with you; he will never leave you nor forsake you" (Deuteronomy 31:6, NIV).

Thank you, Linda, for showing so many how to live...and how to die. See you in heaven, my friend, basking in the presence of our precious Savior. I'm also thinking about a brisk walk on a clear morning in glory. Together.

Joni Eareckson Tada

DEDICATION

*T*O MY DAD, KARL, WHO TAUGHT ME that when girls put their minds to it, they really can do anything that boys can do, and that true strength comes not from hiding our fears and tears, but in letting them out for everyone to witness.

To my Mom, Bonnie, who gave me life the first time around, who taught and then showed me that every cloud does have a silver lining. She sacrificed part of her own body to give me a chance to see more of those special clouds and make a difference with the second go-around.

To my sister, Karen, who proved that sometimes your best friend is just down the hall in your own home, that horror movies are always best when watched with someone else, and that if I just trusted God and her I really could see *Through the Darkness* and experience a realm of life that very few people have the blessing to know. Thank you for making the mall a true adventure!

To my best friend, husband and the one man I am certain was and is <u>the</u> only man God meant for me. Greg, I have loved you for more than three-quarters of my life. Thank you for taking the leap of faith to share a life with me. Many would have leapt right back out when the going got rough. Others would have felt they had bitten off way more than any one man could chew. You, however, have shown me and countless others what it is to be a real man—brave solid and strong—yet compassionate and sensitive too. You have truly made my life an amazing, safe, exciting and beautiful place. You are the main reason I fight so hard to live. You will be a part of my soul forever. Thank you, Boo!

We have been given the ability to have emotions and the capacity for higher thoughts so that we might cry for those things that hurt us, desire things that wash us, and yearn for that which brings us closer to God. We are given tears so that we can cleanse ourselves and move on in a better, maybe stronger, way.

Linda Nordyke Hambleton

God made man
  because He loves good stories.

                    ~ Elie Wiesel

The End
of the
White Picket Fence   1

I'M HAPPIEST WHEN I WAKE UP BREATHING. I am acutely aware of the exchange of air through the lungs, the pulsating movement of blood in a vein, the billions of electric impulses that form a thought in the mind. Life is an amazing gift.

There was a time—long ago—when such things were taken for granted. Somewhere, on the edge of my memory, I can vaguely recall days when these activities took place unnoticed and unappreciated. It was a time when my body served me like a faithful assistant: It took me where I wanted to go; it did what I asked; and it communicated what I wanted to say. It was a short season when my body functioned more or less without effort—days when superficial whims and desires could nudge me to and fro. I was healthy; my soul free, my thoughts drifting like a toy boat dancing with the breeze.

And then it all evaporated like a mirage in the desert of reality.

Yes, I am happiest when I wake up breathing. But today, each breath has a price; each hour costs; each day is expensive. Today the blood still pulsates, but every beat of my heart depends on a delicate balance of needles and pills. Each day is a complex series of steps in an intricate dance to maintain life—a dance that my doctors, family and I share together. The breathing continues, but basic bodily functions are sustained by machines, a sacrificial family, and teams of medical experts. Thoughts still form in my brain, but they are focused and strategic since clear thinking is necessary for physical survival now. And when it comes time to move, every movement is preceded by careful planning and a concerted, intentional, conscious focus of my will. A growing percentage of my day (much more than half now) is spent in bed, in pain and, at times . . . in fear.

"Life" is an amazing gift. I am more convinced of that now than ever before. But as M. Scott Peck wrote in the opening words of *The Road Less Traveled*:

Life is difficult.

Pollsters and census takers make a living by trying to describe life with numbers. Some of those statistics look like this:

- ✧ 234,000 people live in Orlando, my hometown.
- ✧ The average family has 2.37 kids. (My family had only 2.00.)
- ✧ 128,000,000 Americans suffer from a chronic, degenerative disease.

✧ 250,000,000 people in the world have diabetes, as I do.

✧ Seven to ten percent of those diabetics have type I diabetes, as I do. The rest have type 2 or pre-diabetes.

✧ Approximately 16,000,000 people in the Unites States don't know they have diabetes . . . yet.

✧ . . . and 100 percent of us face death, many of us every day.

Certainly, simple numbers cannot define us, yet the statistics that describe our lives have a story to tell. Here are a few of mine:

Since contracting my disease, I have experienced:

✧ 128 hospitalizations

✧ 6.75 average days per hospitalization

✧ 37,500 shots

✧ Two organ transplants

✧ 69-74 pills/day, or about 168,000 total

✧ 2 heart attacks

✧ 3 cardiac arrests

✧ 3 strokes

✧ 250+ grand mal seizures and about 150 focal seizures

✧ 12,000 laser blasts to my eyes

✧ 52 inches of incisions, 255 stitches and 137 titanium staples

. . . And then there were the three minutes that I was clinically dead—but that's for later in the story.

When it comes down to it, however, there is really only one statistic that matters: *I have been given one more day.* Just one more day. Over and over I am reminded that there are no guarantees for tomorrow—and if today is all I have, I have both the opportunity and the responsibility to embrace it, to experience it and to invest it in something that matters. By God's grace, when I wake up breathing, I know that I have been given one more gift, another moment of time to touch, to heal, to celebrate, and to love.

Each molecule of oxygen that passes through my lips reminds me that I'm living in a moment suspended between the temporary and the eternal. Another minute, another second, is not guaranteed. Someday our moments on this earth *will* end. In the Bible we are told to "number our days" so that we might have a "heart of wisdom" (Psalm 90:12). Someday each of our stories will be punctuated with a final period. It's not a matter of if, only a matter of when.

Between now and then we can expect a life full of laughter and tears, joy and grief, struggles and freedom. I guess that's just part of the human condition. The ups and downs are dealt in different measure at different times as the road of life takes us across stunning mountain tops and descends into deep and dark valleys. Together we share a common sense of concern, urgency, disillusionment, and the hopeless cavern of despair. Is there anyone who will be spared "the dark night of the soul"? I don't think so. Undoubtedly, life *is* an amazing gift and life *is* difficult . . . for *all* of us.

Frederick Buechner once said, "My assumption is that the story of any one of us is in some measure the story of us all." Yes, every human being shares a common journey, a walk through this thing called life. The details differ, of course. Our starting points and end points look completely unique. The bumps and potholes jar us in individual ways. The major detours from our desired path show great variety. Yet common to each one of us are a handful of experiences that make our stories the same: basic expectations, broken dreams, familiar fears that assault us, and the looming shadow of death that seems to follow us everywhere we go.

That, I believe, brings us to one of the central and most pivotal points of human existence: What do we do when the darkness descends on our lives? Where do we turn when difficulties and pain threaten to snuff out any sense of light? Difficult circumstances bring us to moment-by-moment decisions—critical junctions in life's journey. At these crossroads choices must be made. They are places where truth must be embraced, laughter must resound above silent despair, and where peace with our Creator and Lord must somehow be harmonized with the glaring realities of difficult worldly circumstances.

But I'm getting ahead of myself already. Allow me to backtrack a little (Let's go back to where it all began . . .).

I was born on July 11, 1965. I would like to think that I was special to someone besides my mom, dad, and grandparents. I'd like to say that my birth somehow shook the world. As they tell it, however, I had a rather unremarkable entrance into the sea of humanity. My little body was absorbed into the billions of others without fanfare.

While America tried to navigate through the tumultuous

years of Vietnam, Woodstock, and the British invasion of rock 'n' roll, I soaked in the security, love and comfort of a strong nuclear family in a typical middle-class suburban home.

My dad: kind, devoted, faithful and strong—unquestionably strong—and not just strong when I need him the most, but strong all the time (because we always need him). He's honest too, particularly with his feelings. His tears and his laughter are never far beneath his professional exterior. He's the one who can make me smile no matter how tough things

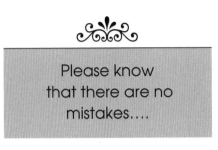

Please know that there are no mistakes....

seem to be. My mom: quiet, poised and elegant, never seeking the spotlight. She is far, far stronger than her delicate body lets on. She feels deeply too, but sometimes she's almost clinical about the challenges that we face. Where Dad might dissolve into a slush of tears or laughter, she chooses to not waste energy on what can't be changed—always focusing on what can be done to genuinely help. And then there is my sister, the little sister who is a sibling and became my first best friend, protector, confidante, and my eyes. Mom, Dad, and Karen—three individuals, but one force of love that are inseparable from who I am, intertwined with the memories of the fabric of life.

I sometimes wonder where those first memories of life really originate; it's hard to tell sometimes. We share so many stories around our home that I can't always discern my memories from stories others have told over and over. Memories of past Christmases, for example, come back to me like snapshots—faded Polaroids, but still sharp and clear in my mind. When I hear "Christmas" I see pictures of gifts, lights, trees, and laughter with grandparents, aunts, uncles, and cousins. The adult figures seem to be permanent fixtures in time and in our hearts, cemented in our souls with traditions like Grandma's Christmas Eve angel food cake coated with a thick layer of white icing. From the small nativity crèche in the living room, she borrowed Mary, Joseph, and the baby Jesus and placed them on the cake. When she carried it to the table, we erupted in song, singing Happy Birthday to Jesus. (We've done that ever since I can remember, and every year it touches me—like a link in the chain of our family history that connects us to that first Christmas over two thousand years ago, when God gave the most valuable of gifts—His only Son.

After dessert Grandpa would push away his chair from the head of the table and all would become very quiet. Pulling something from his pocket or opening a book, he read. We never knew for sure what was coming. Something he had found in a book, perhaps. Maybe a poem or something he had read in a magazine—but always something to make me think and make me cry—timeless traditions that became the time of our life because it was life; I could feel it. Because of Christmas I learned to celebrate life, an experience that has served me well through the decades. Without knowing it, I was taught that life itself is a gift, that each day is a present. I was intuitively absorbing how to savor each day, indulge in it, and embrace it, seeing each moment as a simple blessing, both beautiful and powerful.

Did I fully appreciate those days for what they were? I don't think so. I wasn't ungrateful; I was just fairly unaware of the precious things we shared. But true life is made up of contrasts. Gifts are gifts because they fill a void . . . blessings are blessings because they contrast the emptiness of a curse. Life is filled with them all: gifts and voids, blessings and curses.

I didn't know that back then. We children were raw diamonds who had yet to feel the strategic cut of the jeweler, gold ore that had yet to melt within the furnace of the refinery. Christmas suspended us in eternity. Everything seemed fixed and immortal and easy and good. In a child's mind it all seemed entirely permanent . . . as if nothing could or would change. It never even crossed my mind that such bliss was temporary.

My mom makes the angel food cake for dessert on Christmas day now. And my dad has taken Grandpa's place at the end of the table, sharing stories for the next generation.

Yet, for a while, for a brief season on the edge of my memory, I existed in a perfect childish picture of what life was supposed to be. I am an adult now, yet in so many ways, still a child. I want Christmas like that again; I want the past back with Grandma and Grandpa Early and all we shared. I was living in a Norman Rockwell painting . . . complete with the proverbial white picket fence.

A single routine appointment with the doctor would change all that.

March 9, 1972: Not an unusual day in the history of the world. Nor was it an unusual day for the Nordyke family. Dad was at work; Mom was ticking off items on her never-ending to-do list. One of the things on that list was a visit to our doctor—a "well visit" they called it—a routine annual checkup to confirm what we thought we already knew: I was healthy and happy. But this doctor, unlike most doctors, did a urinalysis as part of his routine. Just a little awkwardness as I peed in a cup and gave it to the office nurse. Done. No big deal. We got in the car and moved on to the next item on the to-do list.

Mom was the one who took the call that evening. It was the doctor's office; they wanted to do more tests. "What are you looking for?" Mom asked. "We need to do some more tests," they said. "We need to do one more."

Every breath, every heartbeat, every thought . . . I have learned to embrace each day as I used to seize each of my presents piled under the Christmas trees of childhood.

The next day's to-do list was adjusted, squeezing in a trip to the hospital. My veins were pricked and poked and I had to swallow this awful orange liquid—so thick it made me gag. "It's a glucose tolerance test," they told us (words that sounded ominous but had no meaning to a six year-old-child).

That afternoon we waited in the hospital for news. Finally the doctor's nurse asked both my mom and my dad to meet him at his office. My parents arrived. The doctor shut the door and asked them to have a seat.

"Please know that there is no mistake . . . ."

It was the end of the white picket fence.

Life is an amazing gift.

Life is difficult.

My body is battered, inside and out. Most "normal" people would be aghast to know the illness and trauma every organ and body part has endured; outwardly, at this point, only those who know me and love me see beyond the physical debilitation that has left me scarred, tethered to IVs and machines, and nearly immobile. But I'm beautiful—perfect, God says so, and I am awash and radiant in fragrant love from the very amazing, caring, devoted people in my life. My heart is weak but full of gratitude. When I add up all the blessings, I find the grace to realize that my serious chronic disease has actually contributed to my incredibly wonderful, beautiful, and exciting life. Most normal people (or, should I say, relatively healthy people) might be aghast at that, too.

Every breath, every heartbeat, every thought . . . I have learned to embrace each day as I used to seize each of my presents piled under the Christmas trees of childhood. Each was mysterious, given with intention, waiting to be unwrapped and savored. Unlike that sheltered, childhood bubble, though, I learned to savor each day when the taste is sweet, bittersweet— or just very bitter . . . sometimes so bitter that all the sweetness seems to have been boiled out of the prognosis for life.

Life is a gift. Life is difficult, too, and disheartening, disillusioning, discouraging, and dark, sometimes very dark. I know, I've been there; I am there. And because my story is your story and your story is my story, I sincerely believe that together we can share an ongoing discovery of a gift that brings unquenchable light into the corners of the deepest shadows:

The defiant candle of hope—a bending, dancing flame that flickers alone—rebelling against the storm of broken expectations, pain and death.

You and I were created for joy, and if we miss it, we miss the reason for our existence . . . if our joy is honest joy, it must somehow be congruous with human tragedy. This is the test of joy's integrity: is it compatible with pain? Only the heart that hurts has a right to joy.

~ Louis Smedes

Once we truly know that life is difficult—once we truly understand and accept it—then life is no longer difficult. Because once it has been accepted, the fact that life is difficult no longer matters.

~ M. Scott Peck

The First Needle

*T*HE GRAPEFRUIT SEEMED SO OUT OF PLACE in the sterile room, sitting on the table next to the syringe. It was March 10, 1972. Outside the hospital the din of life continued as usual. To the casual observer that day looked just like any other day in Cleveland, Ohio: men in huge bellbottomed pants, women with fishnet leggings, children going about their assignments at school with peace signs on their tie-dyed T-shirts. Men were blowing each other to bits in Vietnam and politicians casting blame for it in Washington . . . all the normal stuff. From the viewpoint of space, the earth appeared to be revolving on its axis as it slowly arched around the sun, just as it always had. But it wasn't.

Inside the hospital the world had stopped rotating, hanging dead in its orbit. The man in the white coat told my mom and dad that their little girl was not just their little girl—she was a "juvenile diabetic." My parents sat in stunned silence. The news seemed so foreign—as if it was coming from a strange source, meant for someone else. My mom took me in for a *well* visit. I was happy, healthy, with no particular symptoms whatsoever. We had no history of the disease in our family. None of it seemed to compute. (Five generations back one of my relatives had had diabetes, but that was so far back that the chance of my condition being genetically linked was basically zero.) In spite of what the doctor said, maybe this *was* a mistake . . . .

The needle went into my leg . . . the first needle. It felt like a pinch really, but this pinch sent shockwaves through my soul. I was scared, crying . . . *am I dying?*

Diabetes is not an overly difficult disease to understand. Sugar is one of the main fuels for the human body and it is carried in the blood. The human body is both an elegant and fragile machine. Like most of its requirements, sugar levels need to be regulated within a narrow band of concentrations. Too little or too much blood sugar can cause immediate as well as long-term damage. It's the job of the pancreas to maintain these blood sugar levels with a biochemical called insulin. The doctor told my parents that my pancreas no longer produced insulin to keep my blood sugar in check.

As it turns out, a bad case of chickenpox seven months before my diagnosis might have been the cause. The chickenpox virus looks very similar to the insulin-producing cells in the pancreas. It's possible that as my body fought off chickenpox, it also destroyed my insulin-producing cells. We will never know for certain. What we did know that day was that something serious had invaded our family.

Experts say that the human heart goes through five stages when it faces stunning loss or difficulty:[2]

✧ *Denial* of reality.

✧ *Bargaining* with God (or other authorities) to change the situation or diagnosis.

✧ *Anger* when it appears that nothing can be done.

✧ *Depression* if the anger is not dealt with.

✧ *Acceptance* as the heart embraces the new reality and begins to adjust expectations and actions accordingly.

We didn't have time to deny anything. Nothing had changed; but everything had changed. All looked just as it had the day before . . . the day before we got the call. How could one man's words alter so much? We hadn't asked for life to change. We were doing just fine as we were, thank you. The doctor didn't offer the disease to us with the option to "take it or leave it." He didn't give us an evening to "sleep on it and then call back in the morning." It was simple, but so confusing. We felt like we had just driven into a thick fog: One moment we were cruising along the road of life enjoying the ride and soaking in the view, then, whoosh, just like that, the windshield went gray. While we tried to figure it all out, we still had to keep control of the car. (Denial, bargaining, anger, and depression would just have to wait.) We had to accept where we were and we had to act . . . immediately.

And that explains the grapefruit and the syringe on the table in the sterile room.

The skin of a grapefruit, we were told, has about the same feel and thickness as the flesh of my leg. The syringe is necessary to deliver life-sustaining insulin to the body. We needed to learn to inject the insulin into my flesh. It was the beginning of a new ritual for life:

- ✦ Draw back on the syringe plunger to the volume of insulin required.
- ✦ Insert the needle into the vial and push in the air.
- ✦ Remove the required amount of insulin + five units.
- ✦ Flick or tap on the syringe to allow the air bubbles to rise to the top.
- ✦ Carefully expel any excess air and insulin.
- ✦ Pull the needle out of the vial.
- ✦ Choose a fleshy spot on the back upper arm(s), upper thigh, buttocks, or middle to lower abdomen.
- ✦ Clean well with a swab or cotton ball and alcohol.
- ✦ Insert the needle into the flesh (straight or at an angle—it's a personal choice).
- ✦ Draw back to make sure no blood appears.
- ✦ Depress the plunger to inject the insulin.
- ✦ Continue to live.

First we practiced on the grapefruit. Then I got my first whiff of an alcohol swab and its cool touch on my skin. The needle went into my leg . . . the first needle. It felt like a pinch really, but this pinch sent shockwaves through my soul. I was scared, crying . . . *am I dying?*

The fog thickened. Maybe it was the tears, maybe it was my mind; all I know is that it was very blurry that day inside that hospital. The big words that the doctors and nurses used and the comfort and fear coming from my parents' uncertain expressions were more than my six-year-old mind could absorb.

The nurses gave the first shots. When my dad gave me the next one, it became foggier still. My dad, my comforter, my protector . . . was hurting my body . . . none of this made sense. More confusion: *How many times do I have to do this? I'm just sick. Sick people take shots and get better. Won't I get better?*

I asked my dad a simple question (one that a six-year-old should never have to ask). My dad gave a simple answer (one that a father should never have to give):

> "Daddy, what will happen if I don't take my shots?"
> "Honey, if you don't you will die."
> "Okay," I said. I dried my tears and I never questioned the syringe again.

The first needle. In a surreal and significant way, I began living that day. Deep within my heart the needle made some sort of a connection with my soul, awakening it to the fact that I really did exist. The syringe and all it symbolized gave me a new conscious awareness, telling me who I was, opening up my little childhood world to larger perceptions. I certainly couldn't have put words to it back then, but that day I began to see that life extended beyond my own little childish horizons. I had joined the ranks of multitudes of people who had been awakened from the slumber of superficial life by "the call."

The call comes in many forms. A lump found in a breast, blood in the urine, a spot on an X-ray, a sharp pain in the chest,

a bruise that won't go away, frequent urination . . . sometimes
it turns out to be nothing. Sometimes the doctor asks you to
come to his office, closes the door and asks you to sit down.

The call, be it from broken expectations, broken bones, or the
sting of a needle in a bewildered child's leg, must eventually be
accepted—and even embraced. The stages of denial, bargaining,
and anger are all part of the journey into real life. Author and
speaker Tim Hansel fell while mountain climbing. It was a simple
slip that catapulted his existence into chronic, incurable physical
agony. He wrote:

> *PAIN. It seems to be the common denominator of our
> human existence. It's part of the life experience. To avoid
> it is to detour the essence of life itself.*[3]

. . . The essence of life itself . . . When *the call* comes, assump-
tions and expectations halt dead in their tracks, as if the very
rules of existence have suddenly changed. Everything looks
different. Things unnoticed become vivid. Priorities that
seemed so important evaporate. Things that we thought were
real (that we can touch and feel) turn out to be just mirages.
The true substances of life (that can be neither counted nor
measured) become tangible. Life can be smelled, tasted, and
touched for the first time. Often a rainbow of emotion descends in all its colors.

At least that's what happened for us. When we left the hospital, we entered this new essence of life itself, even though
everything looked the same.

For me this new life was pretty simple: *Pee on a strip of
paper. Drop a tablet in a test tube with pee in it. Take a shot. Don't
even think about asking for popsicles and cookies again.* That was
it. That was life as a child diabetic.

For the adults around me, my disease was much more complicated and much more scary. Diabetes is an ongoing balancing act—a continual shifting of numbers and molecules that must be kept within the narrow range that makes life possible. Sometimes after playing hard I would fall asleep or become very lethargic. I often became obstinate and cranky and weepy. My rollercoaster attitude seemed like an emotional thing, but it was a physical thing. I found it increasingly difficult to understand and concentrate in school. These were just a few changes that my family and teachers had to learn to deal with.

I have found faith in a forgiving, loving God to be an absolutely indispensable necessity— as vital for life as the oxygen in my lungs or the blood in my veins.

As we got our bearings, the earth began to spin again, sort of. On the surface my days were filled with friends, school, activities, and a family that deeply loved me. But they gave me a special kind of attention, attention that gave me a strange sense of being different—and being different is rarely a friend of the child. The teachers had a special note from my parents telling them about just how different things were now, just how different I was now. Between peeing constantly, needing sugar when my level was low (skipping out mentally when it was), and drinking as if I'd just returned from a long trip to the nearest desert, this was the new normal.

We had to watch sugar levels in my urine very closely back then (this was before they were measured in the blood at home; blood sugar testing was only available in the hospital labs), so I had to go to the bathroom a lot. The other kids noticed. I needed to be around people who could respond in an emergency, so slumber parties were out of the question. My feelings were amplified through my new self-consciousness. Often I felt like the odd duck—that I was the only one, that I was alone. It was my first experience with being called a name for something I had no control over, something I did not ask for, something that made me feel funny sometimes and self-conscious always. And then having to take all those shots . . . all the time. I was hoping the mean name-callers would grow out of it just as much as I was wishing I would eventually grow out of this diabetes thing.

Things changed some in eighth grade when a boy from my class walked up behind me and asked, "You have diabetes?" The question flustered me. (Someone had dared to break into my little world, to expose my little secret.) Part of me felt invaded, even a little offended. "Why, does something show?" I responded both insecurely and with a hint of sarcasm. "No, no," he said. "I saw you giving yourself a shot. I do that too."

He gave himself shots? I was fascinated! Here I was at thirteen meeting my first fellow diabetic. I'll be forever grateful that Brock broke the ice that day. Sure, I was different. Sure, there were only two of us, but for the first time I was different with someone else. We had our own little special club which, understandably, no one else seemed to want to join.

Disease has the power to change. But no disease has the power to change a greater, more powerful force—puppy love.

My family moved to Orlando when I was ten. Within the first

few days at Sabal Point Elementary, I laid eyes on this incredibly cute, toe-headed boy. I mean, he had the blondest hair and most perfect lips I had ever seen. Hmmm, those lips just looked like they wanted to be kissed. I started doing what any wide-eyed, giggly, ten-year-old girl with a crush would do: I started writing letters and he started writing back. The paper-based relationship grew and grew as our letters were delivered back and forth by fellow classmates. Finally, on Sadie Hawkins day, I wrote a letter that finally popped *the* question: Will-you-go-with-me? (Nobody was sure what "go with me" really meant, but just the sound of the words made me feel tingly all over.) For convenience I included the classic three little boxes where he could check either yes, no, or maybe (just to keep our options open). My heart danced its own little tango when the letter came back with a checkmark decisively in front of *yes*.

> We were learning to live in a world where normal was never normal.

Scandal would soon abound. Our social science class was on the cutting edge of high technology at the time: We had filmstrips, complete with phonograph records that went "Bing!" every time the strip was to be advanced. That's right, filmstrips. That meant the lights were off. One afternoon, with the room glowing from the light cast upon the screen, we watched a filmstrip about the bicentennial of our country. Slowly, the blond boy's fingers wiggled their way toward my hand. Waves of whispers rippled through the room. Children started getting out of their chairs to look across and see if the rumors were true. They were. The new girl and the blond boy were holding hands under the desks.

Awkwardly, we learned the dance of romance. Friends continued to relay written messages. We tried to appear indifferent to the daily brush of our shoulders against each other during the commute between the lunchroom and the playground. We pretended to ignore the touch of our feet while sitting next to each other on the bus during field trips. But every now and then we would steal a few glorious minutes of handholding—always hoping that nobody was looking, always hoping that everyone was.

Young love in the first degree. But how could I be sure it was the real thing? One night at the roller skating rink, I strategically held hands with a brown-haired boy and waited for the news to get back to the blond I really cared about. Let's just say I had a romantically mischievous side. (The blond haired boy, now fully grown, says that "vindictive shrew" might be a more accurate description.) It worked. "I heard you skated with Randy C.," the blond said to me in the hall the next day. "Whatever you've heard is whatever you heard," I responded. Then I turned and left him standing alone. I walked away with the biggest grin on my face; I knew he was jealous and I knew that I had done it. Where did I learn such things as a ten-year-old?

One time I was over at his house watching TV. His mom said, "It's so nice outside, why don't you go out and play or something?!" She didn't specify what "or something" necessarily meant, but when I pasted one on her son's lips I found out in no uncertain terms that "or something" didn't include kissing. Still, I discovered that kissing really sort of kind of was really something . . . and I really sort of kind of really liked it.

At the end of fifth grade, the boy's parents determined that his academic requirements would be better served at a private school. Distance could not deter us, however. I was running around in the street and yard with some friends one day, pretending that I was Lindsay Wagner, the Bionic Woman when my little sister ran over with a piece of paper and a ring from a gumball machine. He wanted to let me know he wasn't quite done with me yet. (I still have that crazy ring somewhere.) In response, I gave him one of the most endearing symbols of pre-adolescent affection—an eraser . . . but not just any eraser, one of those *smelly* erasers. We were that serious; we were gumball-ring and smelly-eraser serious.

I went home one day and told my mother that I was going to marry the blond gumball ring giver. She said, "Sure. Okay honey." But with him moving to a different school, my guess is that she thought I would never see Greg Hambleton again.

Disease, puppy love, and faith—all became new realities during those tender years. I had been raised in a devout home: church, prayer before meals and bed, Sunday school, Vacation Bible School—I never knew life without God in the background. Genuine faith was infused in our family and I don't remember a day I didn't believe. As I walked through adolescence, though, God came out of the background and into the foreground. Dad taught me the Lord's Prayer when I was six years old. In his version, he put an extra "ever" after "forever." The prayer, then, concluded with ". . . forever and ever, Amen." That sounded like a long time to a young child. And I thought about that . . . I still do.

At age thirteen, I was allowed to decide for myself where my commitments and trust would rest. I took classes, studied other religions, and carefully considered my options. But in all honesty, I already knew what I believed: God exists. I am sinful. God came to earth as a man, Jesus, and sacrificed Himself on the cross so that I could be forgiven. I could choose to either reject His forgiveness or accept it. I had chosen to accept it and enter into a personal relationship with Him. I confirmed my faith in this Jesus on April 14, 1977. My parents gave me a sterling silver medallion with the date of my commitment inscribed on one side and my name engraved on the other. My church gave me an adult Bible (leather cover, gold pages . . . the real deal). To some the choice may have seemed like a childish preference—a superficial adherence to a few mottos and worn out religious clichés. I know better. It was important to me back then and it is essential to me now. I have found faith in a forgiving, loving God to be an absolutely indispensable necessity—as vital for life as the oxygen in my lungs or the blood in my veins. I had learned much as a child during those magical Christmas mornings. Confined to a room with a herd of cousins, we were corralled until just past dawn. We knew we wouldn't even get to peek at or open our stockings unless we ate breakfast first, Grandma's slow-cooked, soaked overnight Quaker Oats were turned into a warm bowl of the best oatmeal there was. A glass of milk and orange juice later, the last bite

> If I was to realize those dreams, I knew I was going to have to fight, and I knew I was going to have to hurry. The doctors told my parents I would probably not make it past my twenty-fifth year.

gone, and we got to tear into our stockings. At that point, led by one of the adults, we headed for the living room like race horses. Whoops and hollers shook the whole neighborhood, ribbons and bows and paper flew in a flurry of both greed and gratefulness—all unleashed in childish innocence.

Christmas was, and is still, all about gifts. Even as a child, I was thankful for the gift of the first Christmas and I held God's Son in my hands. Then, on the edge of becoming a woman, I unwrapped the gift and held Jesus tightly to my chest. I knew how much I loved Him but I still had no idea of how much I would need Him. Today, I don't claim to know very much, but I know I have a greater scope and a broader perspective because of the intimacy I have been given with the One who does know all things. Yes, I need Him; I just don't think I know how much yet. That I will know as I draw my last breath.

As the years ticked away we found ourselves in an odd kind of groove. As we continued to learn to live with my disease, nothing seemed to go smoothly and nothing came easily. I guess that was the groove we were getting used to. We were learning to live in a world where normal was never normal. As we coped with daily obstacles, I grew determined to push beyond them . . . and I started to dream *real* dreams—not the whims of impulsive desire, but deep heartfelt yearnings. I began to see three things that I knew I had to have if I were to live a fulfilled life.

✧ First, I wanted to find true love. I asked my endocrinologist, Dr. Crockett, to please keep me alive long enough to get married to a man I truly loved and who truly loved me.

✧ Second, I wanted to have a baby. Maturing maternal desires had mixed with childhood visions of being a mommy, and I wanted to hold a real child—my child—in my arms.

❖ And thirdly, I wanted to experience disease-free living. My memories of diabetes-free childhood were so vague and so far in the past. I wanted to go back there—back to the days when my life was not governed by the syringe and insulin.

After *the call*, I intuitively understood that life doesn't always work out the way we want. I had begun to accept that. And yet I instinctively knew that sometimes life *could* work out the way I wished. I had a disease, yes, but that just made the challenge more obvious and I knew challenges make victories so much more rewarding. Could it be that my disease was, in some odd way, a gift in and of itself?

When Lance Armstrong (the bicycling legend and seven-time winner of the Tour de France) received his cancer diagnosis, a soldier with cancer e-mailed him: "You don't know it yet, but we're the lucky ones."[4] Lance thought this guy must be nuts. Lucky to have a life-threatening disease?

Back in the hospital room in 1972, I didn't feel lucky. The sting of the first needle pierced far too deeply when we first got *the call*. Today I know better. I was one of the lucky ones. I had been awakened to true life. I had breath, I had a heartbeat, and I had dreams. If I was to realize those dreams, I knew I was going to have to fight, and I knew I was going to have to hurry. The doctors told my parents I would probably not make it past my twenty-fifth year.

In the midst of winter, I finally discovered within me an invincible summer.

~ Albert Camas

The trouble with steeling yourself against the harshness of reality is that the same steel that secures your life against being destroyed secures your life also against being opened up and transformed by the holy power that life itself comes from.

~ Frederick Buechner

A Fight
on
Our Hands

3

*T*HE MEDICAL TERM IS "EMESIS"—A DERIVATIVE of the Greek word "emein," which, according to most etymologists, comes from the Indo-European root "wem."

Around our house we just called it barf.

Barf is an involuntary response to something that the body senses is not right, something the body doesn't like, something the body wants to get rid of. It might be the result of strange motion, too much alcohol, chemotherapy—even stress and fear. Put stuff like that in the human body and it will become emetic and "eject the contents of the stomach through the mouth."

Without bragging too much, I have to admit that I'm pretty good at it—but then, I come from a long lineage of ancestors who excelled in the field (or, should I say, expelled in the field). We were coming back from Christmas one year, in the home stretch from a long road trip. My sister and I were exhausted but vocal; my parents were tired. Deep inside I began to sense that familiar churning.

"I don't feel very good," I said.

"Hold on," my dad said nonchalantly.

"Can't," I said.

"Sure you can; only three more blocks. Just hold on, hold on," Dad said.

"Daddy, there are no handles on emesis. Expulsion of upper digestive tract contents is imminent," I said (in not so many words). Then I went emetic all over the back seat of the car.

"You traveled six hundred miles and couldn't hold it another dozen yards?!"

"Told ya," I said.

On another road trip my mom had gotten very sick from food she ate at a Vietnamese refugee camp at Ft. Walton Beach. (That's a story in itself. During the Vietnam War, temporary camps were set up here in the United States for refugees of that vicious conflict. We had just visited one in Florida.) The conditions were awful. The things we saw left a huge impression in my mind . . . and the things we ate made an even bigger impression in Mom's stomach. At one point, Dad tried to open the door for her, but just didn't quite make it in time. She redecorated part of the front seat as well as the entire inside of the passenger side door . . . and did so with all the accompanying sound effects.

"What are you doing, mommy?" Ever curious, my little sister shoved her head between the doorjamb and the headrest trying to get a front-row view of the commotion. I, on the other hand, have a phobia against such things. When one of my senses encounters the smell, sound or sight of a good old emesis, my body basically says, "Monkey see, monkey do!" So while Mom was doing her thing and Karen was inspecting the damage, I crawled to the very back of the car, covered my head with a blanket and a pillow, and screamed at the top of my lungs to further cut out the sounds, smells, and sights.

"Ketoacidosis." Now there's another interesting medical term. Sounds like something Mary Poppins would sing: Supercalifra-galistic-ketoacidosis! Even just the sound of it is simply quite atrocious."

When the body's blood sugar gets out of control, the sugar in the blood becomes acidic. The blood actually becomes poisonous, slowly damaging tissues and organs. Because a diabetic's blood sugar levels often fluctuate outside of healthy levels, we have an ongoing chronic condition that causes slow, ongoing damage to the body.

Ketoacidosis can also become acute (an immediate threat to life). For me, it started with tremendous difficulty breathing, which is not just a physical challenge, but also a mental one— the sensation that I would suffocate in my own skin. To make it worse, every breath I could muster was thick with the smell of ketones, which is like breathing in a room filled with acetone, the paint-thinning solvent—but I couldn't get away from it because it was in me. My head felt like it was stuffed with packing material. I couldn't think or orient myself to my surroundings. My skin and joints hurt and the headaches were phenomenal. Gut-wrenching vomiting ensued, followed by endless dry-heaves as my body tried to get rid of the acid any way it could. I was being attacked from within; with each episode, vital organs were eroded. Even more terrifying was the threat of immediate death. Only massive doses of intravenous insulin could bring my blood sugar back under control, requiring a stay of four to eight days in the hospital.

Even those dark days in the hospital were filled with light, however. Dad sometimes snuck my little sister into the ICU—which was carefully guarded by a nurse who ran that floor like a dictatorship. Dad tucked Karen under a trench coat, concealing her as living contraband to get past the nurses' station. Nurse Nazi never saw my sister coming in, but Dad never bothered to hide her on the way out. I never quite figured out what she thought—seeing my sister leave all the time but never coming in. Maybe not such a stickler, after all. Good people. She was doing her job—keeping me alive. All together, my family and the hospital staff formed an army to fight off the acidic attacks. I started to get to know the hospital staff pretty well between 1977 and 1979 (from age eleven to thirteen), when I had twenty-nine episodes of acute ketoacidosis.

They clicked on the light to find me writhing and thrashing in a bloody lair of shattered glass. Dad knelt down into the mess with his bare knees as I twisted and convulsed, grinding glass into us.

In eighth grade I was diagnosed with another really good tongue twister: mucocutaneous lymph node syndrome. Most people refer to it as Kawasaki's Disease, because a Japanese doctor, Dr. Lee Kawasaki, discovered it. Oh, how I wish it had something to do with motorcycles. This syndrome came on like the German measles—with an extra symptom thrown in: All my skin came off, *all* of it—eyelids, tongue, toenails, even the inside of my private areas. I could peel off hunks of skin from anyplace on my body. I once started peeling at my palm and tore away a continuous sheet of skin all the way up to my elbow. My body was reduced to a raw, exposed chunk of meat—of course, it was excruciating, like a burn patient inside and out.

Dark and difficult days, but from the shadows, God continued to provide what I needed—more fellow soldiers to fight with me and for me. My pediatrician, Dr. Irvin "Tom" Taylor, was definitely one of those. Kawasaki's Disease was so rare that few had even heard about it back then, yet my doctor "just happened" to have been at a seminar describing this syndrome shortly before he saw my symptoms. His awareness of my condition spared months of agony, even my life. Kawasaki's had nothing to do with my diabetes. It was just a bad roll of the dice. In fact, I'm the only diabetic that has ever been diagnosed with it. I'm also the oldest person to get it.

Ketoacidosis was a battle. Kawasaki's was a true fight. Seizures were war. None of us saw them coming; no one knew what to do about it. We didn't even know what a seizure was, but within six months of the first needle, they began to assault me.

For me, seizures attacked without warning and retreated without memory. Time evaporated in between. I couldn't remember a thing. For my parents, however, each seizure was a nonstop blur of activity. Dad did his best to hold me down and keep me from hurting myself while Mom prepared a glucagon shot to get my sugar levels back up. Twice Dad put his hand in my mouth to keep me from biting off my tongue. I bit his fingers down to the bone instead. (He got a tetanus shot for one of them. The human mouth has a lot of bacteria and the doctor recommended that Dad let the dog bite him next time . . . fewer germs.)

Mom developed a sixth sense about when I was in danger. Maybe it was the mother-daughter connection; maybe it was an angel. All we know is that at night, when I would start to seize, Mom would "hear" the phone or doorbell ring, jolting her awake. It was like God's alarm clock telling her to wake up and rush to my room. Oftentimes she would arrive just as I was beginning to go into a seizure, just before I began thrashing out of control.

Seizures basically fry the brain for a short period time. Each time I regained consciousness, it felt like a huge buzz—a light-headed sensation that was followed by a terrible sense that something was wrong, but I didn't know what. I heard voices, "Chew, honey, chew. Now swallow please . . . ." My brain could hear Mom and Dad, but the words seemed so strange to me. *Why do they keep talking like this? Don't they know that I'm here?* But I wasn't really there; I was somewhere deep inside fighting to get out, as if my soul was asleep somewhere inside the body, trapped and insulated.

"What happened? What's going on?" I would ask.

"Honey, it's okay. You had another seizure," Dad would say. "It's okay."

But it wasn't okay and we all knew it. As the comatose feelings in my head dissolved, they were replaced with uncontrolled sobbing. It had happened again; my body had betrayed me.

I was flooded with the sense of being absolutely and completely out of control. I didn't get a warning; treason came from nowhere. Epileptics have their share of seizures, too, but they usually see little sparkly lights or smell something strange before it happens. I didn't get anything, and believe it or not, that made me jealous; at least they got a few moments of warning.

My parents became seasoned soldiers working together in the midst of the battle zone, which was sometimes just brutal. One night, sensing that my blood sugars were a little bit low, I went downstairs to make myself a sandwich. Somewhere between the open refrigerator door and the counter I fell into a grand mal seizure. I dropped the sandwich and the Corelle plate. (Those plates don't break; they shatter into about a thousand and one pieces, really tiny slivers and shards.) My parents heard the commotion and ran downstairs. They clicked on the light to find me writhing and thrashing in a bloody lair of shattered glass. Dad knelt down into the mess with his bare knees as I twisted and convulsed, grinding glass into us.

In the ER, as the nurses picked glass out of both of us, Dad made light of it immediately. "Honey, the next time you make a baloney sandwich, just use a paper plate, okay?" It was just another little bump in the road. For me it was another graphic picture of my dad: My protector, defender and hero, willing to enter my war, sacrifice himself for me time and time again. Between 1981 and 1983, I had more than fifty full-blown grand mal seizures.

Merle Shain said, "There are only two ways to approach life—as a victim or as a gallant fighter—and you must decide if you want to act or react."[6] I suppose we could have raised the white flag and rolled over on our backs and called it quits. But we couldn't. We intuitively knew that we had to fight. We just had to; and shortly after I turned sixteen, I found someone who truly understood what I was going through. As I got to know her she became my companion—a comrade who has stood by my side and who has led me through many, many personal battles. I didn't find her in the hospital, and I didn't find her at school. In fact, I've never met her. She became my friend through a book.

Joni Eareckson Tada suffered a broken neck in a swimming accident at the age of fourteen. In her autobiography, *Joni*, I found not only a model of hope, but also a mentor, someone in the trenches with me. Her road to physical, emotional, and mental stability was a vicious one—a rainbow of emotions, thoughts, and experiences as she restructured her life around the reality of being a quadriplegic. Our stories are different. A single accident violently shocked her body with devastating and immediate paralysis. My disease works more patiently, slowly eating away at my body just a little at a time. But the core battle is really the same—as it is for all of us—it's a battle for the heart. In Joni Eareckson Tada I found a tale of honesty and transparency and a vision of victory in the soul that supersedes anything that may or may not happen to the body.

When I picked up her book, I had never read a grown-up inspirational autobiography before. As the story of her journey unfolded, I was energized, empowered, even fired up! I wanted my life's story to read like hers; I wanted to be a warrior. Yes, I wanted to *survive*, but after reading Joni's book, I knew that I also needed to *thrive*. I wanted to keep my dreams alive. I wanted to be a model and a mentor to others, just as she had been to me. I wanted to encourage people to fight for life in a war that is physical, mental, and spiritual. I wanted to help people find the light of hope in their dark places.

Fight or flight? Victor or victim? Life's course is largely determined by choice. I'm not in denial here; I know that there are certain physical limitations to our existence that must be recognized. I also believe that these limitations need to be challenged. When hardship and difficulty come, they need to be looked squarely in the eye and told, "Do your worst. This will not end without a fight." The fight for life, fueled by hope, is what makes life worth living in the first place. As Tim Hansel said:

> *I believe that pain and suffering can either be a prison or a prism. The tests of life are not to break us but to make us. We are called not to flinch from real trouble, for the greater part of life occurs in the inner man.*[7]

A dramatic accident, a chronic degenerative disease, or any other kind of tragedy (even those that aren't physical) demand confrontation. They are just asking for it. Staging a successful fight requires picking out essential tools for the battle. Information is one. When I was diagnosed, the only real information we received was in a pamphlet that looked like a child's comic book; in fact, it was a child's booklet with animated images, elementary language, and very simple analogies to describe my disease. It said that the body runs on sugar like a car runs on gas. When blood sugar is low, it's like all the gas is gone. When there's too much gas, you need the help of insulin to get it back down.

That was all the info we were given. My parents and I knew that we were facing a serious life-threatening condition, but we really had no idea what to do. We just knew that there was an enemy lurking out there and we had no idea how to really identify it or to defend ourselves against it. Lack of information is never good, particularly when life is in balance. It's okay to have high blood sugar now and then, but when blood sugar levels are low, brain damage is imminent, as is death. If sugar levels are too high, vital organs are compromised. The booklet didn't disclose the incredible importance of understanding certain facets of diabetes and dealing with them immediately. It was hit-and-miss for about six years.

Finally my parents took me to see Dr. Hulda Wohltmann, a pediatric endocrinologist at the Medical University of South Carolina. She worked with my mom and me every day for two weeks. She walked us through everything. When my mom and I left, we were floating on cloud nine. We finally felt like we had some sort of control; we had a battle plan.

If we had gotten educated earlier, things may have turned out differently in the long run for me. How many brain cells had I killed through low blood sugars and seizures? How many kidney cells did I destroy with high blood sugar? I'll never know. I do know that there's no excuse for that today. Information matters and information is available. That's the reason I'm so excited about the new Florida Hospital Diabetes Institute. This institute will save thousands of lives just through education. On top of that it will offer first-rate state-of-the-art care that will help many, many others avoid the types of complications that I've had.

A basic understanding of diabetes and a willingness to implement some basic lifestyle changes *drastically* reduces the chances of someone getting Type II diabetes and can significantly improve the quality of life for those who already have it. It doesn't matter what the disease or injury, *information and education are critical.* The amount of information available today is astounding. It can even be overwhelming at first, but every bit of information helps to make informed, involved choices.

During those early years I also learned that no soldier fights alone in this world. The team of people that God has put around me, the comrades that fight with me side-by-side, they are unbelievable blessings: They keep me alive and they keep me wanting to live. I'm surrounded by men and women who have exceptional personal and professional skills. Some are brilliant scholars and physicians. To them I owe my life.

> When hardship and difficulty come, they need to be looked squarely in the eye and told, "Do your worst. This will not end without a fight."

I've learned to trust them—but not completely. The people of the medical community are, after all, just people. They overlook things. They make mistakes. They certainly don't know everything. I've learned to ask lots of questions, to get second opinions and seek out alternate explanations. I've also learned to say, "Thank you, but I'm going somewhere else."

I'm convinced I have the best parents and sister in the entire universe, yet they, too, are human. Their capacity to love me and sacrifice for me is mind boggling. But, like everyone, they have their off days. Men and women are not gods. We only have one of those . . . one God . . . the one the Bible calls the "Great Physician." Trust in Him is the overriding aspect of all life. The way that God provides for me through other people sincerely takes my breath away. I don't deserve what I have been given; their commitment to me defies any logical explanation. A greater love works through them toward me. When I say my prayers I give thanks, for I know where that greater love ultimately comes from.

Each soldier must choose to fight, but again, none fight alone. Certain kinds of physical challenges require help; they just do. The illusion of self-sufficient and independent life is really just that, an illusion. Deep dependency links us together as humans. A debilitating condition awakens us to the fact that life is not a solo sport; it simply cannot be played by an individual. The day that my father told me I had to take my insulin shots or die, he also told me something that I've never forgotten. He said, "I promise you, Linda, you will always have insulin. You'll never have to worry about that."

Dad has gone to great lengths to live up to his promise. One Christmas we were making the annual road trip to Grandma and Grandpa's house. The car was basically packed from dome light to floorboards—like the closets in cartoon homes that explode when someone opens the door. The time came for my shot. I was looking for my insulin everywhere and couldn't find it anywhere in that car. Dad quickly dropped us off at a motel in Memphis. As he pulled from the parking lot, two men ran from a liquor store across the street and then disappeared into the night. Dad didn't think much of it and drove like mad through the city trying to find a pharmacy that could sell us what we needed. When he got back to the motel, the police were everywhere. The liquor store had been robbed; two people had been killed. When Dad told them what he had seen, the police were angry that he hadn't stopped when it happened. If he had, however, three people could have been dead on the scene, not just two.

The only reason I'm here today is because Dad, Mom, and a team of others are dedicated to keep the breathing going, the heart beating, the thoughts thinking. I have no question in my mind where I would be without them. In emergency situations, quick action has saved my life many, many times.

Through it all we have learned to laugh, I mean really laugh. At our dinner table, it didn't matter how stressful or how heavy the day had been, we were always spouting off ridiculous jokes. Dad even allowed his two "princess daughters" to use some rather off-color language to spice up our slightly over-the-edge humor. I guess he figured that if we purged four letter words out of our system at home we would be less likely to have them leak out during class. Mom just rolled her eyes and pretended not to hear.

Humor helps; it just does. And not just people laughing *with* me, sometimes they have the sadistic audacity to laugh *at* me. Karen, my little sister, does this all the time. When I'm bedridden and in terrible pain, I can count on Karen to come into the hospital room and say something like, "Hey, want to get up and play some Uno? Maybe dance or something?" Once, after I had just had abdominal surgery, she started cracking silly jokes and saying stupid, sarcastic things—something about me being a pin cushion with miles of zippers. I can't tell you how bad it hurt to laugh. I almost popped a string of stitches.

It's strange to laugh in the face of such serious life situations. I'm not even sure why it's funny at all. E. B. White, the author of *Winnie the Pooh*, said, "Analyzing humor is like dissecting a frog. Few people are interested, and it's bad for the frog's health." Bad for frogs maybe, but as a person moves out of denial and toward acceptance of a condition, I don't think laughter is an option; it's a requirement.

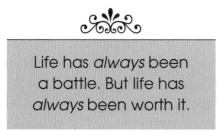

Life has *always* been a battle. But life has *always* been worth it.

Christopher Reeve, the Superman-turned-ventilator-dependent-quadriplegic, said, "My injury gave me firsthand knowledge that humor is also one of the best ways—if not *the* best way—to channel anger . . . . Most of my efforts were rather pathetic, but they were still necessary to ease frustration and manage anger . . . . Sometimes I would pull up to a door and then bark like a dog to be let out . . . . Jokes about the wheelchair helped defuse my anger about being in one . . . . one of the highlights after my injury was Robin Williams' sudden appearance in the ICU dressed in full scrubs, impersonating a manic Russian proctologist."[8]

Chris Fonseca, a Mexican comedian with cerebral palsy, tells about the day he started choking in a restaurant. He frantically waved his hands to get someone's attention. "Wouldn't you know it, I accidentally proposed to a deaf girl! So I'm married now."

Laughter in the face of personal tragedy? Some might feel like that's inappropriate, insensitive, or rude; but, then again they're not in our shoes. I think humor is a great act of defiance against the things that attack us. Laughter is flashing the middle finger at the pain and agony of disease and injury. Good humor is built on a foundation of love with no intention of demeaning the one who suffers. When someone loves you, they can make fun of your situation, your disability, your disfigurement, because they love you beyond the adversity. They mock the ailment while communicating love and acceptance. There's a fine line there, I know, but I believe that as long as caring motives are clear, there is no need to hold back.

Jill Kilnmont, for example, was paralyzed in a skiing accident. In her autobiography, *The Other Side of the Mountain*, she recalls the early days when everyone was trying to pamper her and pretend like nothing had happened. When a brash young boyfriend came over for dinner, Jill asked him to cut her meat. "Ah, cut it yourself," he retorted and kept on talking about himself. Jill started laughing, but the family was shocked. He had the guts to sit down next to her quadriplegia make a joke about it? Yes—and he wasn't being insensitive; he was fighting for her. He validated her as a person when he acknowledged the reality of her condition, shrugged his shoulders, put his thumbs in his ears, stuck out his tongue, and said "tbttbtbt-tbtbt" to her paralysis.

When the dad of one of my friends was dying of cancer, the disease drained him from 230 to 135 pounds—leaving a jaundiced walking skeleton of his former self. In the mornings, while the family ate breakfast, he would come out onto the landing in front of his bedroom in his boxer shorts and pretend he was a body builder—flexing like Mr. Universe but looking like a prisoner from a concentration camp. The family laughed so hard they choked on their cornflakes.

Laughter and humor are indispensable weapons for the battle. Yes, sometimes laughter is the best medicine.

The teen years ticked away. There were quite a number of hospitalizations. Some were serious and some just a little less than serious. While I was fighting *for* life, I never forgot to *savor* life. Perhaps because life was so costly, I could see the value of each day in a special way. Taking each moment into my heart and milking it for all it was worth, I celebrated the days—never quite sure what was around the corner. Though each day was a celebration, Christmas continued to be the pinnacle of the year. The traditions, the flurry of giving and receiving, the hours of loving and laughing. I thought it would go on forever; an island of permanence in the raging sea of change.

Christmas Eve always climaxed with a table filled with family and food; Grandpa always sitting at the head and Grandma always at the foot. In between, our constantly growing and shifting family filled every space. When we were full of food and laughter and stories, Grandpa would push back from the table and read the story of Christmas Eve from his Bible. Together we held hands, sang one verse of a favorite Christmas carol, and thanked God for the celebration that lie ahead.

Sometimes the traditions of old were spiced up in unexpected ways. The year I turned fourteen we were Christmas caroling as a family. We rang a doorbell at random, and when it opened, I found myself looking at the blond-haired boy— the boy who was no longer a boy, but who was yet to be a man. A sixty- second dance in adolescent awkwardness ensued: not acknowledging each other's presence, but fully aware of it; no eye contact, but seeing each other perfectly; not a word spoken between us, but communicating loud and clear. By all outward appearances, the chance encounter was a non-event, but neither of us ever forgot it.

"Fighting while savoring" is a strange balancing act. Having grown up on this crazy teeter-totter of disease I've never known anything different. Life has always been a battle. Life has *always* been worth it. Gathering information, learning how to give and receive as part of the team, seasoning every serving of life with as much humor as I could, learning to laugh at everything from barf to ketones, from seizures to tears—it's all part of the journey. Perhaps Alexander Pope captured the paradox best when he said, "You purchase pain with all that joy can give and die of nothing but a rage to live."[9]

I was in an ongoing fight to live. I had "a rage to live" and I could see that the fight was worthwhile. Or so I thought. We had learned to dance in the fog and celebrate in the rays of sun that always seemed to permeate the clouds somewhere. Little did I know that the darkest days were still ahead.

Literally.

You do not have to sit outside in the dark. If, however, you want to look at the stars, you'll find that darkness is required. The stars neither require it nor demand it.

~ Annie Dillard

Blind Faith 4

*T*HE OPHTHALMOLOGIST SAID, "DON'T WORRY ABOUT IT. You're just a teenager. All young people think they need glasses; it's kind of a fashion statement. Just stop over-focusing and it'll be fine."

"Okay," we said.

I heard the doctor's blunt and condescending words, but I wasn't sure what they meant. What did he mean by over-focusing? Focusing was my problem. I was squinting all the time, sometimes even seeing double. My parents nodded and I didn't feel it was my place to question him. He was, I was told, a specialist in diabetes. We accepted his analysis and did what he said: We didn't worry about it.

It was 1983 and I had just graduated early from Norcross High School in Norcross, Georgia. That fall we moved back to Orlando where I started school at the University of Central Florida. Early in January, however, my roller coaster health took a significant dip. My attendance in classes was erratic at best, continually interrupted by health issues. In early February I was admitted to the hospital with significant abdominal pain and bloating. The doctors decided to take a peek inside with a laparoscope to see if there was a mass or tumor that might be causing the pain. They put a mask over my face and I descended into the gray of unconsciousness via general anesthesia.

Coming out from under anesthesia is always a blurry experience—so hard to tell what's real and what's not. That day, as I waited for the blur to clear, my brain hung out in limbo, looking for something tangible to grab onto. When I tried to get up, I almost passed out, and the nurses put me back in bed for a little more rest. When I opened my eyes again, however, everything was very silvery, kind of like looking through crinkly, translucent, metallic tissue paper. I rubbed my eyes to make sure that they were actually open. Was I conscious? I was. Everything seemed to be awake, except my eyes. *Maybe it's just night time. That's it; it's just two or three in the morning and the anesthesia is playing tricks on me.* Not so. It was the middle of the day and the sun was shining in my window. I waved my hand in front of my eyes. *Nothing. Nothing.* Fear washed over me. Panicked, calling out for my mom, my dad, for anyone. My dad was there, and when I told him I couldn't see anything, it didn't quite register. I said again, "I can't see anything!" My dad ran into the hallway and yelled for help. Nurses and doctors descended in a flurry of white coats and clipboards. The ophthalmologist took a look and called it "edema of the retina." But he said that if I just took it easy for a few weeks the swelling would go down. "Don't worry about it," he said.

This time, we worried about it. My parents knew something wasn't right. (I thank God that they have always been incredibly proactive in my care.) They called Dr. Wohltmann, the pediatric endocrinologist from MUSC in Charleston. When she heard my symptoms, she told us to drive to Chadeste and she would get us an appointment with Dr. Gerre K. Chambers, the head of the Storm Eye Institute at MUSC. She offered me her mother's apartment if one was not available when we arrived. I was alone with Dr. Wohltmann for a few moments before we saw the doctor. She became very sober and very serious. "I have to tell you, Linda, I don't know what to expect. You've got the worst case of proliferative retinopathy I have ever observed."

Dr. Chambers took one look and made his diagnosis.

"We need to start the treatment as soon as possible. I believe some sight can be restored through laser surgery."

"When do you want to start?" Mom asked.

Dr. Chambers said, "I'll be ready in five minutes."

Dr. Chambers used quick blasts of the most intense YAG laser light available—a device that was still somewhat experimental at the time. The laser bursts cauterized (i.e., singed) the active vessels that were bleeding into the vitreous humor (the fluid behind the eye that holds everything in place and keeps it moist from the inside out.) The lasers were the easy part. First, my eyes had to be paralyzed to stop any movement during surgery that might cause the laser to fry the optic nerve or anything else by accident. (If that happened it was all over— all sight would permanently be lost.) Paralyzing the eye required a needle, but not the kind I was used to. It was about three inches long and very thick, inserted through the soft pocket of skin underneath the eye and pushed in until it was behind my eye, and then the cement-like substance was injected, paralyzing the nerves and the muscles.

"This is going to be incredibly painful, but I will only have to do it once," Dr. Chambers said. He was right. It *was* incredibly painful—pain of an entirely different kind—pain from some universe outside of this world. It was by far the most focused, intense pain I had ever, ever felt.

But Dr. Chambers was wrong, too. The first needle didn't do the job. He had to do it *twice*. Another needle. Another wave of indescribable, foreign pain. Finally, he started in with the laser, one thousand blasts to the back of each eye.

It was the beginning of a new routine that demanded time and complete re-arrangement of my family's logistics. The drive from Orlando to Charleston took about six hours each way. The expenses for travel, lodging, and the procedures were astronomical. And all for what? It just didn't seem possible that something that hurt this badly could actually be good for me. I cried a lot; my parents cried a lot. Every molecule in my body screamed in protest as I voluntarily subjected it to repeated blasts of torture. Instinctively my flesh recoiled at the pain of the shots. The anticipation of the repeated procedures required that my mind be stronger than my instincts; I had to consciously choose brutal short-term sacrifice to keep alive the dream of long-term improved health. If I lost sight of the future, every cell in my body would have been relieved to surrender and remain in the darkness. But I wanted to see again. So we made the drive, the doctor inserted the needles, the laser blasted away, and then I would go home.

I did this fourteen times—10,000 miles, 28 needles, and 14,000 blasts of the laser.

The darkness continued. I clung to the hope of light over the next horizon, but the realities of blindness became a new day-to-day challenge. Moment by moment I was forced to face a new level of dependency. Thank God dependable people surrounded me. Karen, my younger sister, became a surrogate set of eyes. Her voice became my radar. "Step up, step down, a crack in the floor...." Her creativity became my confidence. She even taught me how to shop by smell. Arm in arm we walked through the mall, stopping and taking deep breaths at each location. On the next trip, she would quiz me to see if I could name where we were. It didn't take long to figure out. When I needed to get to a certain store, I could just follow my nose.

Karen was my self-proclaimed "seeing-eye-person;" she was my protector. I dated a guy for a while that Karen just couldn't stand. He didn't take care of me like she knew he should. One night we all went out to get something to eat. He got out of the car, didn't bother to open my door, and left me alone in the parking lot—as if I was supposed to walk into the restaurant by myself without any help. Karen was furious. "What are you thinking? What are you going to do, leave her there? Go get my sister!" Then she said, "Never mind, I'll do it." She led me into the restaurant, sat down between us and refused to let him touch me. (She was awesome—like a mother lion with her cubs.)

"I hope you never see him again. He's a jerk." Karen said. I halfheartedly agreed. Inside, however, I felt desperate to have a boyfriend, to be normal, and to feel things that other teenage girls felt. I was only eighteen and willing to take just about anything from any guy to get that. I felt like I was damaged goods. *Who's going to want to date a blind girl with this many problems from diabetes? Who would want me?* My mom and my sister tried to set me straight. I heard them out and believed them to a certain extent, but doubt and rejection still swirled in my heart. I knew my family accepted me, but outside the doors of my house was a different story. How could I compete in a world that judges by appearances, performance, and possessions?

Control issues were powerful. The struggle for independence compelled me. I learned how to read Braille in two weeks (a task that normally takes months). I was desperate to read all by myself, trying to find something I could do alone. Karen learned Braille with me. She could see the raised dots on the paper and quickly memorized the alphabet. We were given a Braille typewriter and Karen used it to catalog all of my music albums and 45s. We used to type letters to each other that were loaded with cuss words—laughing our heads off while my mom and dad were blissfully unaware. It was sisterhood at its very finest: Unity born of adversity; personal bonds that can only be forged in foxholes during battle. Karen started doing that when she was just thirteen. She was truly an amazing kid, but she exuded the grace of an adult.

> Inside, however, I felt desperate to have a boyfriend, to be normal, and to feel things that other teenage girls felt. I was only eighteen and willing to take just about anything from any guy to get that. I felt like I was damaged goods.

My dad, on the other hand, rearranged the furniture. I had done my best to memorize the layout of the house, but he liked to move his chair around in the living room so that he could see the television better. Sometimes he wouldn't put it back, turning my life into a living Helen Keller joke. *How did Helen Keller burn her face? She answered the iron. How did she get blis-*

ters on her fingers? She tried to read the waffle maker. How did her parents punish her? They rearranged the furniture . . . just like my dad. I'd be walking through the room, minding my own business, and all of a sudden, wham! I'd slam right into his chair. Then, from Dad's bedroom I'd hear, "Whoa! Soooooooooorrrrrrrrrrrrrry!" followed by a sinister snicker. I was constant entertainment. I stubbed more toes and ran into more doorjambs than I could ever count. I'd try to dress myself and come out looking like the Grand Champion for junior high "Tacky Day." When we were out shopping, my family would lead me in and out of the clothes racks, but I'd still inevitably bump into one. "Oh, sorry, Ma'am," I'd say. They thought this was hysterical, but I got back at them when we went out to eat.

Forks and spoons are extremely difficult to use when you can't see. We would be out in some fancy restaurant and I'd get frustrated pretty fast—it's hard to enjoy a meal when your spoon forces mashed potatoes up your nose and your fork keeps stabbing your cheek. "Ah, forget it," I'd say, and just pick up my food, pull it apart, and shove it into my mouth.

I laughed a lot on the outside, but hurt a lot on the inside. A lot of people do not know how to deal with people's handicaps, and I felt increasingly isolated from my peers. Still, God had His way of showing me that I wasn't alone. Students from a church that I didn't even attend decided to send me a get well card, just to let me know that they were praying for me and thinking about me. One of the members of the group, Malcolm, wrote a beautiful letter, complete with encouraging Bible verses. One day he showed up at my house with a tape player and a cassette of his favorite Christian artist.

He sounded nice enough, but I braced myself. *Church music? The only church music I know is my mom's stuff that's over 300 years old.* My stereotypes evaporated the moment he pressed the play button. *This is my kind of music! Like the Eagles and Styx.* Even more importantly, the words from David Meece's song, "We Are The Reason," resonated with my faith and my growing need to be loved. They reminded me that Jesus had given His life; that He had suffered and died . . . that He had given all He had to give, for me.

Both the music and its message touched something deep within my heart. In the darkness I was forced to listen, and listen well to what God said to me through this song. A new sense of clarity descended as the truth about who I was and what Christ had done for me reverberated through the music.

Truth, however, is a double-edged sword. The lyrics spoke of love, but a sacrificial love, a love that required suffering and death. This was *true* love, passion mixed with blood, a gift of life shrouded in a human sacrifice. I was standing on the edge of a multifaceted faith; my childish faith was stepping over the edge into a more mature belief—a belief that said nothing real can come from something superficial, a realization that said there can be no light unless there is also darkness.

Before I knew it, Malcolm and I were dating. I could not have asked for a more thoughtful gentleman. He was a gentle and solid guide as I walked through the darkness. Malcolm could see through my handicaps, neither ignoring nor dwelling on my physical struggles. He filled my syringes and gave me shots. He always carried glucose tablets in his pocket. He was a natural. With him I learned to be comfortable with myself. I felt safe with this young man both physically and emotionally. Soon my affections began to swell.

Mind you, I'd never seen him. Yes, I felt his face 5,000 times and memorized the contour of his nose, eyes, and his mustache. But for two years I loved him not knowing what he looked like. And he loved me knowing what I did look like: Two white eye patches under big black glasses, walking into walls, and introducing myself to mannequins. I was a real piece of work.

Malcolm gave me a glimmer of the real thing, a real love. But in time, the glimmer died down, slowly ebbing away like grains of sand washed away by the continuous lapping of waves. Both of us cried the night that we broke up; we both felt it—but what a gift of God he was to me during that most insecure season of my life. I was twenty years old. Wasn't I supposed to be in some sorority surrounded by friends, or wasn't I supposed to be throwing up at a fraternity party somewhere? Instead I was alone in the darkness of my room, wondering if I could ever be attractive to anyone, if I would ever be desired by anyone, if I would ever belong to anyone. Through Malcolm, God's hope flickered again. Perhaps the dream to find true love wasn't out of the question. God was providing for me, indirectly through others like Malcolm and my sister. Beyond that, through a simple song, I was learning that God's direct love was all that and more.

One of the great blessings (as well as the obvious curse) of pain and difficulty is that it brings other aspects of life into vibrant focus. In the darkness my other senses came alive. I was learning to walk by smell, touch, and sound. Without sight I was forced to "see" beyond my circumstances, and I gained a new awareness of life through other senses. Perhaps even more importantly, I was forced to stop, think, and ponder life beyond the visual. In my soul, I was learning to walk by faith, not by sight.

That next Christmas was another traditional flood of sounds, smells, and physical sensation. A grand mixture of celebration and the Savior all blended together in an extraordinary sensory experience. Certainly, there were things that I missed: something silly that somebody wore, the sparkle of a gift of jewelry, or a cute new sweater. But somehow, the "picture" of Christmas actually became more vivid when I couldn't see it. This new "handicap" brought other aspects of life into vivid focus like never before—the smell of the tree, the kiss of a loved one, the children's laugher, Grandma's voice calling from the kitchen. I soaked it all in, able to sense it in new ways. What a mistake it would have been to have missed even one moment of those precious days; what a tragedy it would have been to have lost the vision of Christmas simply because I couldn't see.

Despite Dr. Chambers' assurances that I would regain some of my sight, darkness was still my only reality and I started to hate it—not so much for what it had done to me, but for the way blindness changed the way others related to me. Karen and I would go shopping at the mall and salespeople would come up to me and yell, "Can we sell you something!?" as if I was deaf as well as blind. Everyone, it seemed, talked down to me, using short sentences and little words, as if I was stupid because I had patches on my eyes.

I practiced simple skills that I needed to function in public, hoping that nobody would know I was blind. I wasn't ashamed of it, but it seemed like everyone else was ashamed for me. I hated being different and identified as weak. I didn't want people to pity me. I hated that. I would so much rather have someone say, "I am so sorry you're going through this," and then treat me like a normal human being. Instead, they communicated, "Oh, you poor thing!" *Poor thing?* I have *never* been "poor" and I hated it when people thought of me that way (still do!). I didn't want people to pity me as a little sickly, helpless person. That's not who I am.

> It was like people thought the blindness or diabetes was contagious and if they hung around me too long they were going to catch something. I was a leper, outcast, judged. Some of my best friends slowly faded out of the picture.

Even my close friendships became awkward and strained. An uncomfortable, invisible wall formed between us. Simple comments like, "Hey, good to see you," or "Wow, look at that!" suddenly had them uncomfortable and stuttering all over themselves. "Oh, sorry Linda, ah, I mean, ah, I know you can't 'see' or 'look', so sorry." It was like people thought the blindness or diabetes was contagious and if they hung around me too long they were going to catch something. I was a leper, outcast, judged. Some of my best friends slowly faded out of the picture. It felt like betrayal of the deepest kind; it was pain—another *new* kind of pain, just as real as the needles in the eye, but even worse. The pain of perceived rejection attacks the soul rather than the body.

In the midst of all this, the trips to Charleston continued. Both the blood from the retinopathy and the laser blasts were polluting the fluid behind my eyes, requiring a surgery called a vitrectomy. Dr. Chambers made numerous incisions in my eyes, inserted four to six delicate instruments, drained the blood-infused fluid from the back of my eyes and replaced it with a new artificial fluid.

To relieve some stress and to try to gain some sense of control in the darkness, I did about an hour's worth of exercise in my room every day—full-blown aerobics, jumping up and down—all the stuff that made Richard Simmons and Jane Fonda rich. That was my daily routine until I had an appointment with Dr. Chambers and he informed me that I was not to do any type of exercise. He didn't even want me to shake my head to indicate yes or no. I was shocked. I had no idea I could have blinded myself over something silly and stupid. I was relieved that I hadn't hurt myself. But now, added to the pain and the darkness, was a new sense of fear.

In the recovery room after my second vitrectomy, I knew I was suffering from low blood sugar. Against all post-op protocol, one of the surgical techs gave me grape juice. I vomited violently. When I looked up the world was twisted and distorted—almost like I was looking at a mirror image—like I had an eye on the outside that was looking in—like I could see what was going on even though I was blind. The force of the vomiting ripped through the stitches in my eye and some of the cauterized veins exploded. My eye cavity filled with blood, completely destroying the work that had just been done.

Anger, injustice, and frustration tore through my heart. *Couldn't just one thing go right? Couldn't I get just one little break?* I felt like Job, like I was taking some sort of test that had no answers. *Two steps forward; ten steps back.* Everything that I held to was being ripped away—my health, my friends, my future, my self-image. I know some people struggle to place their faith in the God that they cannot see. I couldn't have seen Him even if He had appeared to me. My new mature belief was pushed to the edge. I tried my hardest, but God just wasn't doing His part. I prayed and prayed for my sight. When that didn't appear to be God's will, I prayed and prayed that I would be able to understand and have the fortitude of faith to get through it without pushing my family beyond their limits.

When I took an honest evaluation of where I was, though, I felt that He had given me neither my sight nor the faith and fortitude to get through the blindness. I was on the edge of blind faith, but I didn't know if I had the will to cross over. Philip Yancey, in his book *Disappointment with God*, captured the core of my struggle:

> . . . *I hesitate to say this, because it is a hard truth and one I do not want to acknowledge, but Job stands as merely the most extreme example of what appears to be a universal law of faith. The kind of faith God values seems to develop best when everything fogs over, when God stays silent, when the fog rolls in.*[11]

I had reached my end. There is light in dark places, *always*; but sometimes it has to be very, very dark to be able to begin to see it.

Vision is the art of seeing things invisible.

~ Jonathan Swift

The God in My Closet

5

*W*HEN EVERYTHING IS DARK, IT DOESN'T MATTER how much light is around you. To someone who is used to sight, the blackness becomes an endless void, a world without definition, an expanse without boundaries, an endless space that leaves you suspended and unprotected.

As the months of blindness added up, the darkness became suffocating. I learned to feel the sun on my cheek and the breeze in my hair, but deep feelings of vulnerability and uncertainty were my constant companion. Large open areas were the worst. I reached out and reached out some more. I took steps and then more steps and still reached out into nothing. *Where am I? Where is the edge?* It felt like . . . like unanswered prayers. If I couldn't grab hold of something and identify it, I didn't know where I was. It freaked me out.

The blackness wrapped itself tightly around my heart, stirring claustrophobic fears. *Who is that in my room? Did I just hear something? What is under my next step?* And it wasn't scary just "out there," it was scary inside, inside my heart. *Who have I become? What does the future look like? What if the lasers don't work? Will I ever find a reason behind this struggle?* I felt that if I could put some sort of purpose to all that was happening I would be able to find direction again. Instead, I felt a menagerie of contradictions in my soul. I needed to be around people, but also needed to be alone. I needed to connect with something or someone to anchor my soul as I drifted in the dark, but I already seemed so isolated.

The "why" question wouldn't rest, either. I began bargaining with God for the things I wanted. I felt I deserved these things for having gone through what I had gone through. *O Dear Lord, I've been through all of these trials and tribulations and I still believe in You. By your grace and mercy please intervene now and free me from this burden.* Inside and out, it didn't seem like things could get worse. And then they did.

I had one friend who had stuck with me, Karen B. (The "B" helped keep her separate from my sister, Karen.) She and I were born within twenty-four hours of each other. From the day we met in sixth grade she felt like my twin. We shared everything we had, every thought, every tear, every dream. We used to write notes back and forth on sheets of notebook paper that we stapled together in volumes. Over the years we accumulated an encyclopedia of hopes and dreams and laughter and thoughts for the future. We were going to do it all together—live together, find husbands together, have kids together. I even dated her brother for a time.

When we were eighteen we vividly dreamed of getting our own apartment. We had the colors picked out. We had the furniture picked out. We even knew the view and location, too. In reality, there wasn't an apartment in existence that met all our qualifications—at least not one that was within a tenth of what we could pay. Together, though, no dream was impossible. Somehow, somewhere, that apartment was going to be ours.

It wasn't to be. A mutual acquaintance of ours became obsessed with Karen. His affections and infatuations seemed flattering at first. Then he began to pursue her in uncomfortable ways. His locker was plastered with her pictures. He kept calling; he kept showing up; he kept asking her to go out with him. She was one of the sweetest and most caring, loving, and generous Christian women that I knew; she wouldn't do anything to hurt anybody. She kept saying no to his advances, insisting that the relationship stay on a friendship level.

He wormed his way in, however, taking advantage of her giving, caring nature. She was a whiz at math; he struggled to pass. He talked her into tutoring. She helped him for several sessions, but his advances became more emphatic. Finally, she drew the line and said no more, but he begged and pleaded for her to come back and help him just one more time, just to get through the exam. He promised that that would be it, he wouldn't ask her out anymore, and he wouldn't bother her again.

Maybe she was just too trusting, maybe too naïve, or maybe she was so sweet that she just couldn't say no like she needed to. I'll never know for sure. What I do know is that on the way home from that final tutoring session, he again asked her to go out. She said *No.* So he took her behind a movie theater, stabbed her to death, and threw her body in a

> Even through this valley I believed God was still there; but did He care? If so, why didn't He do something about what was happening?

dumpster. She was twenty-one.

I was sick and weak when it happened. My parents decided to wait to tell me the news. When I was out of the hospital, Karen's brother, Michael, came over and told me what happened. He had painstakingly prepared an album for me, full of newspaper clippings and paraphernalia from our friendship. Together we wept and talked for hours.

A new flood of questions: *Why? Why? Why, God, did you let this happen to such an incredible person? There are plenty of just awful non-believing, atheist jerks out there that are running around healthy and free. Why her? Why now?* I wanted an immediate answer. I wanted the doorbell to ring, for some angel to be there with the top-ten list of why this happened. I didn't want to wait to discover some subtle lesson. Her life had been taken so fast and brutally; I wanted a fast and brutal answer. The details of her death only made it worse. He didn't just kill her. He purposely hurt her as much as possible before he took her life. I had always watched the news and heard, "So-and-So was murdered . . ." and I would always say "Gosh, I'm glad I'm not so-and-so's friend." Well, guess what? All of a sudden I was.

I felt something snap inside; all the questions that I had suppressed about my own situation broke free and rushed to the surface. I used to hear about people that went blind from diabetes, and I always said, "Gosh, I'm sure glad I'm not one of those people." Well, guess what? All of a sudden I was. *Who am I going to have an apartment with? What happens to all my plans? Who is going to be my special friend now? Why? Why? WHY?* The angel with the answers never showed up at the door. I was left alone in the dark with a huge stack of notebook paper, an album, and a pile of dreams that were never to be. I felt more alone than ever before.

In reality, I was in good company. I had joined the ranks of multitudes of honest people who were asking the honest questions about pain and suffering and finding no answers. Philip Yancey recalls a letter that he received from Meg, a mother who had buried her only son and daughter because of cystic fibrosis. She wrote about her deceased twenty-one-year-old daughter:

> *God, who could have helped, looked down on a young woman devoted to Him, quite willing to die for Him to give Him glory, and decided to sit on His hands and let her death top the horror charts for cystic fibrosis deaths . . . there are moments when my only response is grief and anger as violent as any I have ever known.*[12]

Even King David (whom the Bible calls "a man after God's own heart") struggled openly with his disappointment and frustration toward God:

> Have compassion on me, Lord, for I am weak. Heal me, Lord, for my body is in agony. I am sick at heart. How long, O Lord, until you restore me? . . . I am worn out from sobbing. Every night tears drench my bed; my pillow is wet from weeping. My vision is blurred by grief; my eyes are worn out because of all my enemies.
>
> Psalm 6:2-3, 6-7

Another man, wrestling with his wife's intense chronic neck pain, phrased his frustration this way, "I feel like I'm watching a play being acted out on a stage. The tragedy is taking place, but the hero never shows up to save the day." A more honest paraphrase of all these words might be, "Listen! Don't you get it, God? I'm hurting down here. Where are you? Why don't you do something? Why?"

I've grappled with all those questions and more—though I

never reached the point where I questioned whether or not God existed. I know that plenty of people do that and I sure don't blame them. When things get really bad, it's very easy to question whether or not a good God even exists. I don't have that option; God is just too obvious to me. I know that He *is*, but figuring out what He is *doing* is another story. Even through this valley I believed God was still there; but did He care? If so, why didn't He do something about what was happening?

> The God in my closet was becoming the greatest reality in my here and now, and not just as a newfound *friend*, but as my *Lord*.

I needed something. I didn't need a parent's good advice, I didn't need a well-meaning pastor quoting verses that were borderline cliché, or a counselor trying to sugarcoat what was going on. I needed to be completely real, real with myself and real with God. As vulnerable emotions of uncertainty wracked my body and mind, I knew I needed to find a space, a place that was safe, quiet and definable. I needed a private hide-a-way where I could completely let down my guard, be brutally honest, and let it all out. I found that space in a rather unusual place.

My closet was a walk-in, about six feet deep, maybe five feet wide. Shelves all around, clothes hanging from front to rear—

that thing was jam-packed. I'm not sure what initially drew me in there. I don't know when I realized that this place was small enough to feel safe, yet big enough to breathe. But with my back against the far wall, my fingers caressing the walls on each side of me, I could feel where I was. *Definition. Boundaries. Security. Solitude.* The muffling effects of the clothes softly blanketed all sound from outside. It also absorbed anything that I might say.

I had found my space, the place where I could be completely honest with God without fear of anyone hearing me. I could finally take the lid off my Pandora's Box of emotion. But should I? That is a frightening thought, really. What would happen if my anger and frustration were vented on Him? Would I go too far? Would there be consequences? I was safe from the world in my little space, but was it safe to be honest with God?

I had done some serious searching about anger in the Bible. Was it possible to be *too* honest with God? I couldn't find anything in the Scriptures that suggested this. Instead I found continual encouragement to be open and expressive with Him in both good times and bad. He even commanded me to bring my cares and worries to Him (Psalm 55:22) and to let my tears and frustration out in His presence. Besides, didn't God know everything that was going on in my heart and mind anyway? Wouldn't it have been *dishonest* to pretend that I didn't think and feel the way I did?

I gave it a try. The words came slowly at first, but then I let Him have it all. While the music played in my bedroom, and the clothes absorbed my voice, I got real with the real God. I talked to Him in complete openness, releasing the floodgates of questions and anger that had been dammed up.

I waited for God to punish me for my blatant outburst of raw emotion.

Pause.

No lightning bolts. No worldwide flood.

Somewhere deep in my soul a huge burden was being lifted. I used to think that prayer had to be very formal, like I had to speak in King James verbiage or something so God could understand. I thought that prayer, done properly, fulfilled a formula. *Maybe if I held my hands just right, bowed my head just right, closed my eyes, and spoke in reverent tones, then maybe God would grant my three wishes?* In the closet, I got over that. Prayer sounded more like, "Hey, this sucks. Why don't you fix it?"

When it was all out, when I had dumped everything on Him, I sat quietly, rested, and began to listen. In my secret quiet place, in the stillness around me, He offered no answers, no explanations, no apologies. In a whisper loud and clear He only affirmed that He was there. And that was enough. T.S. Eliot once wrote:

> *To believe in the supernatural is not simply to believe that after living a successful, material, and fairly virtuous life here one will continue to exist in the best possible substitute for this world, or that after living a starved and stunted life here one will be compensated with all the good things that one has gone without: it is simply to believe that the supernatural is the greatest reality here and now.*[13]

The God in my closet was becoming the greatest reality in my here and now, and not just as a newfound *friend*, but as my *Lord*. I felt like Job must have felt when, in the middle of all his struggles and all the lousy advice from his friends, he finally unleashed his frustrations. God responded, "Who are you to question me? Have I not made all that you see? Am I not good and in control of the things that you cannot see and cannot understand?" God was God. He wasn't some errand boy or a fix-it man at my beck and call. He was Lord. He was the Potter and I was the clay. He was the Father and I was the little child. Like a crying newborn, shocked by my exposure to real life, I screamed in legitimate pain and confusion—I had protested because of my inability to grasp the purposes of an infinite, almighty and truly loving Father.

I would have strongly preferred a clear answer to my questions. I would have greatly appreciated Him fixing the dark and difficult circumstances that were consuming life as I knew it. Instead, I received an invitation, an invitation to walk with God and follow Him *through* every difficulty. Jesus said, "I have told you all this so that you may have peace in me. Here on Earth you will have many trials and sorrows. But take heart, because I have overcome the world" (John 16:33). "And be sure of this: I am with you always, even to the end of the age" (Matthew 28:20).

It was the beginning of a different type of relationship with God. Not only could I talk with Him just as I could my best friend, but He was really the *only* person I could talk to openly and without fear. If I was going to have a best friend, who better than God? Who better to share my fears, joys, and dreams? If I was looking for reasons and purpose, why not allow God to be that central focus?

The issue was really about control. I wanted things to work out the way I wanted, particularly things that seemed unjust and unfair. But like it or not, I had to face the fact God really is the one that's in control, I'm not. Fighting for control from God is absolutely anti-productive and, actually, impossible. *Am I really going to manipulate or strong-arm the God of the universe?* Besides that, trying to control things on my own isolates me from the miracles of hope and joy that God can bring about *in the midst* of pain and suffering. He is the one who determines, who orchestrates, who will make all things new and good again . . . someday, in His own timing, for reasons we may never understand this side of the grave. God is constantly orchestrating miracles big and small. By releasing control to God, my eyes can be opened (so to speak) to the way that He works and I can receive the blessings of His miracles in the moment. But the more I fight, the less I see.

When I quieted myself in my closet, the big question wasn't, "Why would God . . . ." It was "Do I trust?" When all hell seemed to be cutting loose, when my whole world felt like it was being ripped out from under me through the horrific loss of my friend, did I trust God or did I not? Personally, I don't believe it's possible for anyone to trust God 100 percent. Anyone who says that they completely trust God in everything no matter what, well, they are lying. (Either that or pain and loss have yet to attack the most important aspects in life.) When the core of our being is threatened, that's when we find out that trust is not something you *have*; trust is something that you *do* moment-by-moment. Trust is a continual ongoing decision in the face of trying circumstances; it is a choice to believe in God's goodness and presence even when He seems to be steering our lives down the wrong path.

> When the core of our being is threatened, that's when we find out that trust is not something you *have*; trust is something that you *do* moment-by-moment.

Yes, it's easy to trust when you don't need to. It's easy to love God when He's doing what you want. But as Frederick Buechner wrote:

To be commanded to love God at all, let alone in the wilderness, is like being commanded to be well when we are sick, to sing for joy when we are dying of thirst, to run when our legs are broken. But this is the first and great commandment nonetheless. Even in the wilderness—especially in the wilderness—you shall love him.[14]

This realization changed everything. I finally made a transition between the "why" question and making a conscious and deliberate choice to trust the God that I loved. The focus of my heart changed from the discouraging and depressing circumstances around me to what I knew to be true about God Himself. Nothing had changed outwardly, but the anger and frustration began to dissipate. While sitting in the closet I had taken a small step and discovered that the smallest mustard seed of faith can move mountains of confusion and conflict from the human heart. Where anger had been, God began to build something different—a heart of thanksgiving. By an act of my will, with that small amount of faith, I was able to talk to Him about the obvious good around me. Then I began to thank Him for the things that I could see no good in, whatsoever. God honored that small seed of faith, and when it was watered with my thanksgiving, it began to grow into something else—peace. When I finally left the closet, I reentered the world cleansed, focused, and more balanced. My circumstances were just as they were when I had entered, but now, after meeting the God in my closet, a peace that surpassed all comprehension was guarding my heart.

I have lost track of how many times I have retreated into the closet. Since those first days I have changed homes twice. Throughout the seasons of life, different kinds of darkness have threatened to snuff out the light of hope in my life. But I always have my closet. It's not always a real physical closet. Wherever I am, I can always find that place of quiet safety, where I can speak my heart openly and naturally before my best friend and my Lord. God Himself promised that if we search for Him with our whole heart, we will find Him. If we knock, He will open the door. As the bumper sticker says: *No God, No Peace. Know God, Know Peace.* By finding Him, I found the peace, and that's really what I had been looking for all along.

I was doing the closet thing one afternoon when my conversation with God kept getting interrupted by words swirling around in my head. I took out a piece of paper and special stencil that had raised lines, allowing me to write with reasonably straight penmanship. I just started scribbling down the words as they came to mind but I ran out of paper. The words were still coming so I turned around and started writing on the back wall of my closet. I didn't know what was going on for sure, but in a few moments the words stopped flowing. Whatever I had done was done.

I wish I could have seen my mom's face when I called her into the closet to see my handiwork. The hesitant quiver in her voice made it clear that she was trying to figure out whether to freak out and go get paint or help me. In her usual fashion, she chose to help. Kneeling in the closet with me, she read the words out loud and together we began to figure out which words went where. She wrote it in longhand, and that evening my dad typed it out for us both:

THROUGH THE DARKNESS

I see many faces in this darkness of mine-
fear, regret, sorrow, pain, and loneliness.
The nightmares seem so real, the days so long.
Sleep comes hard for fear
*   that nightmares will become real.*

Truth is the hardest reality—
in anticipation I see what isn't there.
But, with the love so abundant around me
I also see the face of hope, and it is smiling.

Through the darkness, not around it, not in denial of it . . . *through* it. God was using the pain, suffering and injustice of worldly life to continually draw me back into the closet where I could meet Him in the quietness of safety, honesty, and love. So many questions have yet to be answered. So many tears continue to be shed. But as King David admitted to God in one of his closet poems, "You keep track of all my sorrows. You have collected all my tears in your bottle. You have recorded each one in your book" (Psalm 56:8). The poetry of a man searching for a light of hope in dark places. What did he find? He found that God was close enough to capture his tears in a bottle. To be that close, to be able to catch our tears, means God must be right here, eye to eye, touching our cheek. And when we are face down in despair, God takes the same posture, sharing our grief with us. Dr. Paul Brand wrote:

> *Where is God when it hurts? He is in* you, *the one hurting; not in* it, *the thing that hurts.*[15]

I had broken through. I had sought Him and I had found Him. By a choice of my will, I could now move on.

God is light, and in Him
there is no darkness at all.

~ 1 John 1:5

Endurance is not just the ability to bear
a hard thing, but to turn it into glory.

~ William Barclay

Where There is a Will

6

Major Margaret "Hotlips" Houlihan ran from the shower with nothing on except a towel. Hawkeye Pierce and B.J. Hunnicut poked their heads out of the mess tent trying to smile innocently as ferret-faced Frank Burns chased Margaret toward her tent—only to have the door slammed in his face. I could see it all—in my imagination at least—the actors in army fatigues, the drab green tents on the set, the red and white cross of MASH 4077 on the ambulance. I could see it, but only through my ears as the familiar voices and the canned laughter cut through my darkness.

As I listened to the familiar sounds on the television, I sensed a bug flying in front of my face. *Blind people don't see bugs*, I thought. Indeed, it wasn't a bug; it was a piece of debris floating through the fluid in my eye. This was a regular occurrence. My brain knew it wasn't a bug, but instinctively my hand reached up to swat at it anyway.

A shadow passed through my field of vision.

What was that? I waved my hand again. Another shadow! *I can see?* Hesitantly, I tried it one more time. I passed my hand in front of my face and the shadow again moved through my sight. *I can see!* I slid from my bed and crawled toward the patio and my family. "I can see! I can see!" The exuberance over-flowed. We huddled together like we had just won the Super Bowl, crying and thanking God.

Prior to that day "silverfish" were the only visual sensation I had. When I put pressure on my eyes, it was as if large schools of flashy minnows were swimming in my head. The movement of the shadow of my hand was the first *real* thing I had seen in two years. In the months ahead I began to see little gaps in be-tween the fish where real objects moved in a cloudy blur. My sight *was* getting better. Slowly. Very slowly. Only time would tell how much better it would get, but after the darkness, some sight was certainly better than none.

Amazingly, within about nine months I had functioning, yet very, very fuzzy sight.

A flood of gratefulness rushed through my heart. What I had taken completely for granted was now a precious gift—a gift to complement each breath, each heartbeat, each thought. I had trained my other senses to compensate, but now I had some sight back, too, and life became more vivid and intense than ever before.

I'm not sure anyone can fully appreciate something until it's gone. I had come through the darkness and was moving back into light, a journey that I wanted to capture in writing. While traveling with my family, we stopped at a Kentucky Fried Chicken in Kentucky (how appropriate). Eating mashed pota-toes, I scribbled out new lines of poetry. By the time we got back home to Longwood, Florida, it was done.

INTO THE LIGHT

I have made it through the darkness—mind, heart, body and soul. But I shall not forget from whence I've come. As my eyes grow tired and remember pain, my dreams will keep me humble in thoughts of my struggle to become whole. I regret no more the pain and anguish but hold it up as a symbol that I have made it through the darkness and into the light. (January 5, 1988)

The darkness taught me many priceless lessons and I vowed to never forget them. I had been immersed in nearly three years of deep self-revelation. I discovered what I was made of and what was most important to me. I learned to sit and think for hours at a time. I learned who my friends really were, and I even got to see my friend Malcolm for the first time (turns out he was a pretty handsome guy, though not blond enough for my tastes). Most importantly, in the closet of darkness, I learned how to pray, *really* pray, by walking in an honest moment-by-moment personal relationship with my God.

Perhaps Helen Keller captured the experience most accurately:

If I can get so much pleasure in mere touch, how much more beauty must be revealed in sight? Yet those who have eyes apparently see little. The panorama of color and action which fill the world are taken for granted. It is a great pity that in the world of light the gift of sight is used only as a mere convenience, rather than as a means of adding fullness.[17]

I couldn't agree with Helen Keller more! With a new sense of vision in my eyes and my heart, I made my goal a university degree. While I waited for an opening at the University of Central Florida, I chipped away at classes at Seminole Community College. Each day I faced significant roadblocks because of my medical conditions and blindness. I clung to hope and continued to chip away at my degree assignment by assignment, test by test, class by class.

Meanwhile, my eyesight continued to improve in tediously slow increments. Still, the greatest challenges I faced were not physical, they were mental—the struggle to keep my faith and hope alive. At one point I saw my local ophthalmologist for a routine visit. He said, "I don't think it's ever going to get any better than this. You'll probably never drive again, so don't get your hopes up. "At first, I obeyed the doctor's orders—I didn't get my hopes up—in fact, my hope dissolved with his words. I came home just devastated; that doctor had taken an eraser to my hope. My mom, however, rejected this man's analysis. "No!" she said. "That's not correct. Remember what Dr. Chambers said? We're going to listen to what *he* said. He is fixing this. This *is* going to get better."

Eighteen months later I walked back into that doctor's office with my driver's license in hand. He said he was happy for me—but he said it in the *I-don't-like-to-be-told-I-was-wrong* kind of way. Sticking that license in his face felt mighty good. I was furious that he had almost stolen my most valuable asset: hope. But he had taught me one of my most powerful lessons: Yes, it is very important to be objective and to respond to facts, but interpreting those facts must be done by people who care and are closely involved. I vowed then and there that anyone who was uninformed and uninvolved was not going to be a part of my team or a part of my life—because no one has the right to take away anyone's hope. If you lose hope, you lose your will. If you lose your will, you lose everything. Without hope, I would have had no desire. Without desire, I would not have taken action. Without action, I would have become immobilized, stuck in the mud puddle of pain and discouragement. I simply could not let that happen. No hope . . . no life. It's that simple.

Two and a half years after the MASH moment, my vision correction plateaued. My sight had improved greatly, but it was still horrible by most people's standards (20-100 in one eye, 20-120 in the other). My colors were all mixed up, too. The impulses my eyes sent didn't match up with the colors my brain recognized. I've tried hard to relearn color, but I don't always get it right. That's why other people pick out my clothes now and everyone is much more comfortable when I head out the door with a credit card *and* somebody who has real vision. (No more hunter-green pants and burgundy blouses for me.) Inch by inch I was learning to walk in the light. Amy Carmichael once penned these words in her classic poetic style:

> I vowed then and there that anyone who was uninformed and uninvolved was not going to be a part of my team or a part of my life—because no one has the right to take away anyone's hope.

> *Sometimes when we read the words of those who have been more than conquerors, we feel almost despondent.*

> I feel that I shall never be like that.

> *But they went through step by step*
> *by little bits of wills*

little denials of self
new inward victories
by faithfulness in very little things
they became what they are. No one sees these little hidden
steps. They only see the accomplishment, but even so those
small steps were taken.

There is no sudden triumph
no spiritual maturity
that is the work of the moment.[18]

The closing lines of that poem speak volumes about tenacity. We see tenacity in those who look a challenge in the eye, see that it is worth conquering and, as Winston Churchill said, "Never, never, never give up." Triumph is never sudden; spiritual maturity doesn't appear in a moment. It takes tenacity. One of the gifts of my disease is that if *forces* me to be tenacious. Nothing comes easily. Only by "little bits of wills" am I finding my way and becoming a conqueror.

A fine line exists between tenacity and obsession, however. I discovered that in the college weight room. My workouts started quite normally. It just felt great to exercise—it was therapeutic both physically and mentally. As I pushed my body, I noticed immediate physical results, and I liked what I saw. I finally had something I could control. I may not have been able to control much of what was happening *in* my body, but in the gym I had control *over* the outside of my body. Soon I was working out four hours every day. My biceps grew, my thigh muscles were huge, my neck and shoulders started to look like an Olympic gymnast—a *male* Olympic gymnast. That's when my hunger for control got a little *out* of control.

The more results I saw, the more control I exerted over my body. The more I controlled my body, the better my results. The stronger I felt, the more control I felt I had. The more control I felt, the harder I worked out and the stronger I became. *This was awesome.* It didn't take long before my arms wouldn't fit in my shirts anymore. I kept ripping them at the seams. I started wearing my dad's shirts instead. Pretty soon I morphed into Xena, Warrior Queen Amazon Goddess—a mixture of Linda Evans, the Wonder Woman, and Godzilla.

The guys in the weight room didn't know what to think. Two members of the tennis team were obviously intimidated. (Tennis players have a reputation for being a little bit on the scrawny side anyway; I could have bench pressed both of them at the same time.) One finally had the guts to ask, "Ah, like . . . why do you do this? You know, like, that's really not like all that feminine." I knew deep inside why I was doing it and it didn't involve anybody else. It was for me. It was for control. I had found one thing *I* could make my body do.

Control, however, is really just an illusion. Some things are within our control, but so much of the bigger picture is not. One day on my way home from the gym I turned into a convenience store to get something to drink. Out of nowhere a huge Cadillac slammed into my door. The window shattered, embedding shards of glass into my face, eyes, head, arms, abdomen and thighs. As my car rolled toward a ditch, I grabbed the emergency brake with my right hand and saw a large piece of glass sticking out of my forearm. Within seconds people were everywhere trying to help. When a policeman arrived, he said he was going to call the Lake Mary Volunteer Fire Department. I said "No, no, no. Call the Seminole County Fire Department, Station 35, and tell Sam and Eddie that Linda needs them." It's kind of sad when you're on a first name basis with your paramedics. At least I didn't have my name painted on a parking spot in front of the emergency room . . . yet!

Sam and Eddie arrived, their familiar voices calming my soul. As they assessed my bloody mess I told them about the glass in my eyes. I also told them I couldn't feel my legs; numbness had taken over my body from the hips down. They rushed me to the hospital where a young, green doctor began to stumble through my case, making several initial misjudgments. The doctor insisted, for example, that my eye didn't have any glass in it. Eddie took a Q-tip and rolled my eyelid back and sure enough he found a sizable chunk of glass. Sam and Eddie told me they weren't going to leave me until I got proper help, and they stayed true to those words. Eddie called my parents from the phone at the Nurses' Station . . . I was never out of his sight. Sam was trying to tell the doctor about my diabetes and all the while I was trying to tell all of them that I couldn't feel my legs.

When I was stable, the attention finally turned to the numb appendages sticking out of the end of my torso. I was released from the ER and went to see a neurologist who did an electromyoencephalogram. The results showed that I had no sensory neurological connection between my brain and my legs. I had "drop foot," the blob at the end of my leg hung lifeless as if it had no nerves or muscles. My legs could still receive instructions; they just couldn't do anything on their own.

Using a walker I began going to physical therapy three days a week. At the mall my mom and I would walk (more like a drag-shuffle) from end to end using as much muscle and leg strength as I could muster, always trying to keep that dang foot from dragging uselessly behind me. My workout routine had been reduced from squats with weights to trying to put one foot in front of the other without falling over. After a year I was finally able to walk without tripping or falling—most of the time. The numbness persisted. Even today I can't feel anything from the hips down.

So much for obsessive control.

> *But they went through step by step*
>> *by little bits of wills*
>> *little denials of self*
>> *new inward victories*
>> *by faithfulness in very little things*
>> *they became what they are.*[18]

<hr>

Tenacity toward the university degree never let up. Because of continual interruptions from my health and injuries, I had to take most classes two or three times. One day I was driving to Seminole Community College when a major blood vessel ruptured in my left eye. As the eye fluid began to fill up with blood, it looked as if someone had smeared a thick layer of strawberry jelly across my eye. Then my right eye vision started waning too. I was driving and praying, "Please Dear God, let me get to school in one piece and don't let me kill myself or anybody else along the way!" I made it into the parking lot after running over several cement parking spot markers. I got out of the car and started screaming for help. Jerry, one of my closest friends at Seminole Community College, "just happened" to be walking in the area (another little provision by God in a moment of needy confusion). He heard my voice and ran as fast as he could in my direction. Helping me to the student union, he got me a glass of water, calmed me down and called my mom. Back at home we made the call to Dr. Chambers. When I hung up, I had new things to put in my student planner:

> Dozens of people had selflessly walked beside me, lent me their eyes when I could not see and their legs when I could not walk.

1. Schedule more eye surgery.
2. Inform professors of my two-week absence.
3. Figure out how to make it through school blind.

I had gone blind mid-semester. That meant that I was on the edge of forfeiting all the work that I had already done in my classes. I was most concerned about losing ground in anatomy and physiology, one of the most intense classes of the curriculum. We were ready to take the midterm, which entailed walking around the laboratory and visually identifying specific body parts. With just a sliver of hope, I approached my professor, James Turner, who thoughtfully pondered my plight.

"Let's figure out a way," he said. After thinking about it for a while, he disassembled a full skeleton that he had on display in the classroom. It came apart in pieces like a puzzle. Laying all the parts on the table, he asked me to identify each piece

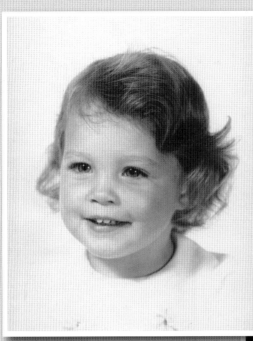

Linda – Easter 1967

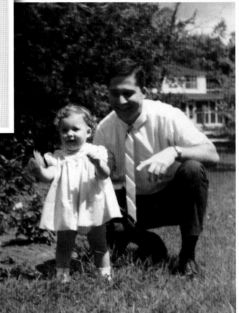

Baptism Day –
hope begins…

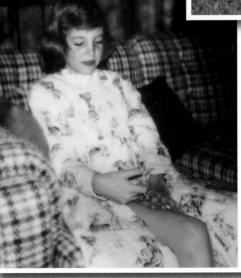

One of 37,500 insulin shots

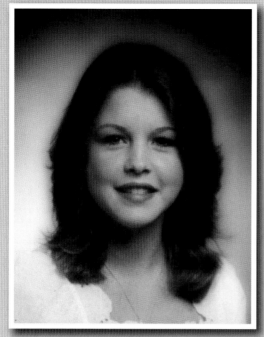

Carefree middle school days

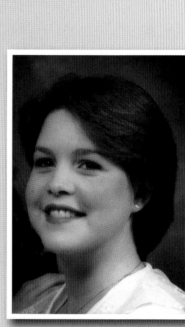

Linda – Sweet 16

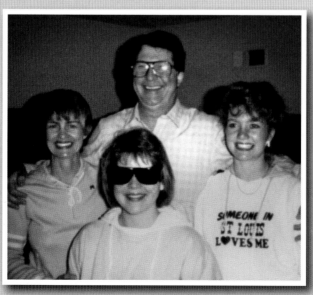

Christmas 1985 – halfway through the
darkness – more eye surgery looms

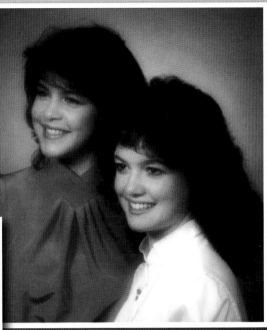

Linda & sister Karen
as teenagers

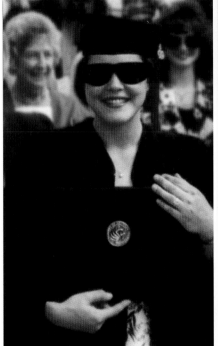

UCF, Graduation Day
May 1992
Mission accomplished!

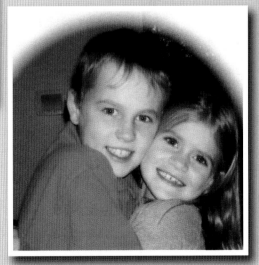

Max & Morgan Palmer
Linda's nephew & niece,
and Junior Prayer Warriors

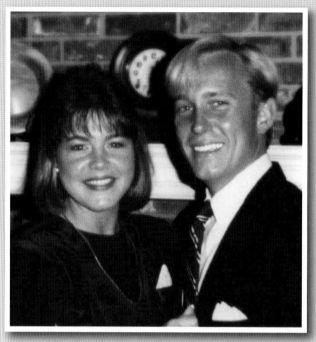

Linda and Greg – July 1988
Love in early bloom

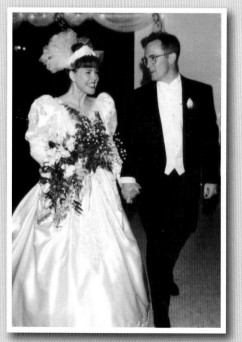

First introduction as
husband and wife

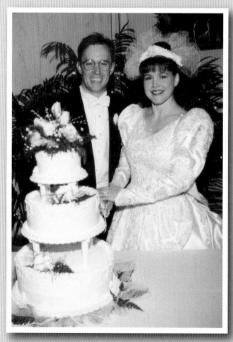

Wedding Day
November 12, 1994

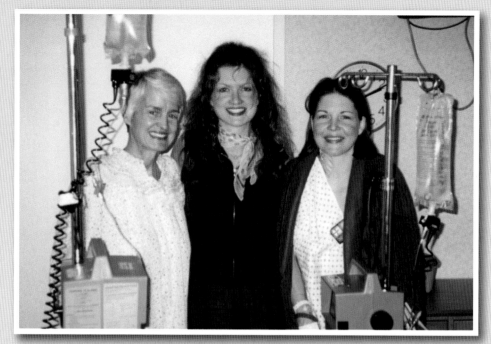

All is well. Linda with her Mom and sister Karen
three days post kidney transplant.

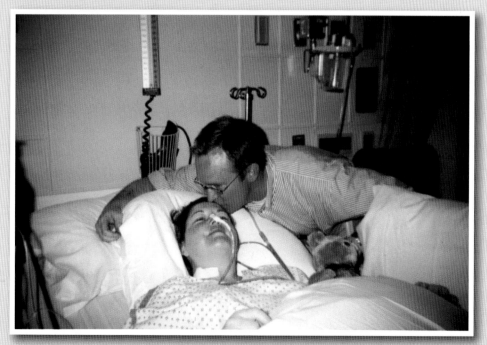

"Babe, I've always got your back."
Taken just after the pancreas transplant

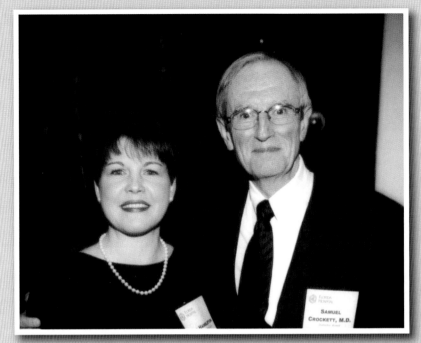

Linda and Dr. Samuel E. Crockett at a
Florida Hospital Foundation dinner

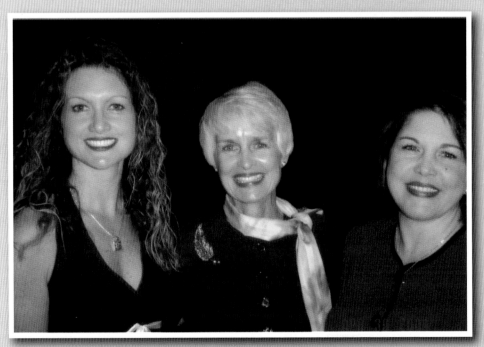

Sister Karen, mother Bonnie, and Linda
at a diabetes fundraiser

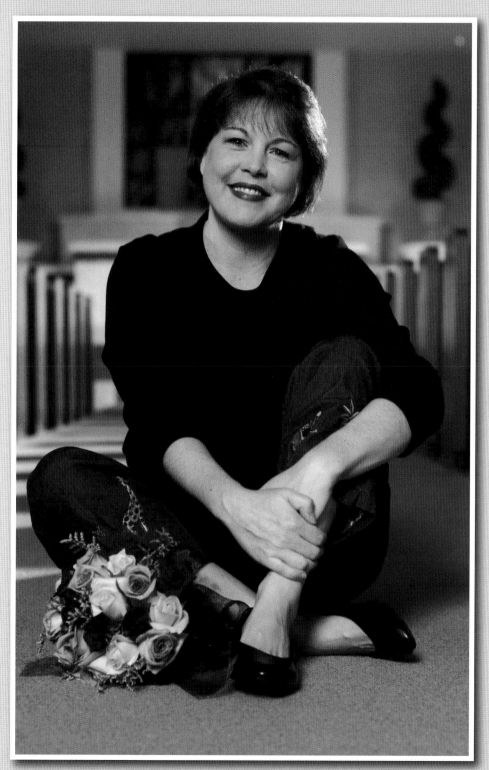

New kidney and pancreas are working fine!
Life is coming up roses.

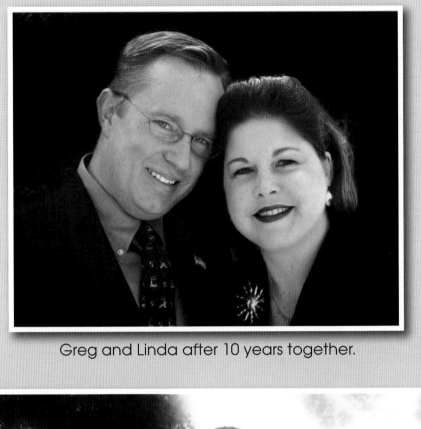

Greg and Linda after 10 years together.

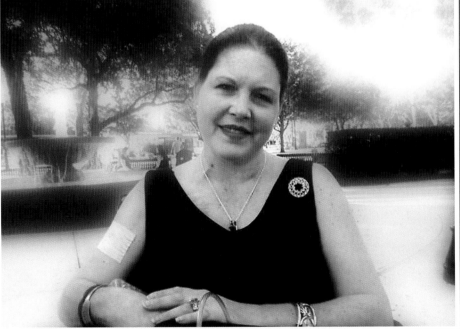

This photo is one of Greg's treasured favorites.
It was their last date and Linda's gaze is clear, serene,
and it conveys love in its purest form.

by feel and describe its function. I did it! The professor was convinced that I had a complete working knowledge of everything that he had taught. I received an A for the class and learned another valuable lesson: Goodhearted people are willing to go the extra mile when they see someone with the willpower to break through struggles. (Thanks, Jim.)

God made some of this much easier, too, by giving me a real knack for certain subjects. I don't like to brag about my academic abilities much (Mom and Dad do enough of that for me), but to be honest, I'm really, really good in math and almost all the sciences—especially if it has to do with medicine. Once, one of my professors wrote a formula up on the board.

"You have fifteen minutes to work it out step by step. When you think you have the answer, let me know."

I raised my hand.

"I'm done," I said immediately.

"Done with what?!" he asked.

I showed him the number I had on my paper. He looked at his sheet, which had a full page of figures and equations. The number that had appeared in my head and the number at the bottom of his paper were the same. He was intrigued! What do you do with a student who can come up with the right answer without working through the problem?

When I went blind, he knew that I had the ability and the determination to do the work, but neither of us was sure how to test it. He turned out to be another person willing to go the extra mile for someone who tried. He created special verbal tests for me and I was able to give him answers without writing anything down.

Absorbing written information was another challenge. My mom and my sister read to me for countless hours, as did faithful friends. I repeated what they read, memorizing it in whole or in part, doing whatever was necessary for the tests.

It worked. All the teamwork and tenacity earned me an Associate of Science degree from Seminole Community College. Next I was on to the University of Central Florida where I had to study through a lot of medication. Sometimes the drugs caused memory lapses. Sometimes I would study all day and night to learn something and then "boom," wake up the next day and it was like I had never even read it. (I know that's common among fellow college students who are unable to recall on Saturday what they did on Friday night, but I think my situation allows for slightly more sympathy.)

Low blood sugars raised havoc with my memory, as well. Random chunks of information just seemed to evaporate. Oftentimes I really needed that information to get through a class. I have a near photographic memory, but sometimes big long strips of the film simply disappeared. Fairly often I would find notes in my own handwriting and have no idea where they came from. I didn't like that at all; it totally freaked me out. That meant there were certain parts of my life that were taking place without me, like I was a total schizo with someone else living in me.

The seizures also continued, and they, too, would wipe out three or four days of memory. Sometimes a block of memory from weeks before a seizure just went "poof." It was so weird, and it was so awkward. I would forget I was at a major event or I would space out an important appointment. More than once my mom and I disagreed about things that she had told me. Stubborn as I am, I would be convinced that she hadn't said anything about it when actually she had. We needed some grace on both sides to get through that.

Quite frankly, I hate the struggles with memory loss. It strikes right at the core of my control issues. It means that precious memories of meaningful events are simply gone. I also had to realize that this was an insurmountable barrier in my career path of choice. My goal was to be either a PhD or an MD. I had the brains, but I didn't have the eyes or the memory. How devastating it could have been to misread a simple prescription or to forget the details of a diagnosis. Practicing medicine was one dream that I had to let go. That was hard. It took a long time to get over (I'm still not sure I have). I was forced to realize that no matter how strong my will might be, physical limitations reduced my options. And that goes for everyone—not just those of us who suffer from a disease or a debilitating accident. On the other hand, we'll have no idea where those limits are unless we push ourselves as far as our bodies and minds will allow.

Where there is a will, there is almost always a way.

"Brick walls are there for a reason. They give us a chance to show how badly we want something."[19]

Randy Pausch wrote that not long before he died of pancreatic cancer. When Randy got *the call* he was already living very intentionally and strategically. But after he received a terminal diagnosis, he quickly accepted the fact that his remaining time on earth was going to be measured in months, not decades. The reality drove him to live not only with a strong will, but also to live in a strong way. Randy's lecture and book, *The Last Lecture*, has deeply challenged our society to rethink their attitude and approach toward life so that when our final day comes, we can look back and know that we held nothing back, we gave it all for the things that are most important. A full life comes not only through the power of will, but through a way of living that embraces a focus and clarity of personal purpose. When we first realize that life is indeed terminal, or when each day is purchased at the price of great pain and struggle, each moment passes with an increased awareness of its value— a value far too precious to live without purpose.

I had graduated not because I was smart, but because I was stubborn.

Lance Armstrong used his bicycle and his fame to create one of the largest cancer research funds. Christopher Reeve spoke to the world through a ventilator to champion the cause of finding a cure for spinal injuries. When each of these men accepted their illness and injury, the next step was to focus outward for causes bigger than themselves. Quadriplegic Joni Eareckson Tada described her moment of realization this way:

> *I was angry that my life had been reduced to the basics of eating, breathing, and sleeping—day in and day out. But what I discovered was that the rest of the human race was in the same boat. Their lives revolve around the same meaningless cycle—except with them, it wasn't as obvious. Peripheral things distracted them from the fact that they were caught on the same treadmill. Their jobs, school, families, and recreation occupied them enough so they never consciously recognized that their lives were the same as mine— eating, breathing, sleeping. Eating, breathing, sleeping. Eating, breathing, sleeping. For what purpose? How can I glorify God? What can I do?*[20]

Pain and hardship, illness and mortality: If we are willing to listen to them they can serve as an alarm clock for our souls, waking us from the slumber of a routine life. Yes, it would have been nice to finally get answers to the "why" question behind my struggles, but when I read Joni's words, I knew that didn't absolve me from the "how" and "what" questions: *How* should my life change because of this struggle? *What* am I supposed to do because of it? I have the will; in what way am I to live it out?

I ask myself those questions on a regular basis. I believe in a God that can take difficult and even evil things and use them for good. How can He use my battered body and my fragmented brain to somehow bring Him glory? Can my story somehow blend with the stories of other people and bring hope and help to those in need? When I draw my last breath—be that in the next minute or in the next millennium—will I be able to look back and know that my life counted for something that really truly mattered?

On August 8, 1992, the president of the University of Central Florida placed a piece of paper in my left hand while he shook my right hand. An indescribable rush of emotions flooded through me.

Relief. The work was over and the stress of papers and tests was a thing of the past.

Pride. I had not only made it, but that I had done so with honors. My degree indicated distinction in math and science. My transcripts showed that I had graduated with a 3.91 GPA. On my gown I wore the tassels of the Gold Key National Honor Society.

Thankfulness. Dozens of people had selflessly walked beside me, lent me their eyes when I could not see and their legs when I could not walk.

And, finally, a tremendous wave of *accomplishment.* Hundreds of students graduated that day and each one had a story, but I can safely say that no one experienced what I did to walk across the stage.

As I accepted that diploma and shook the president's hand, two things went through my mind:

First, I wanted to savor the moment and make it last as long as possible. I was on stage for maybe ten seconds, but each one represented a year of concerted effort. Defying the barriers that stood in front of me, I had simply refused to give up. I had graduated not because I was smart, but because I was stubborn. As I stood on stage, I experienced a sense of focus and satisfaction few others will ever know. Can I be so bold as to say that the pain and the difficulties had enriched the pure essence of life itself? Not the superficial lifestyle of leisure that is so highly esteemed. I experienced the reward of *real* life. I had found a *will* and I had found my *way*, two things that had earned me a university degree with honors; two things that allow me to get out of bed each morning and face the gift of yet another day filled with pain and laughter.

Secondly, I didn't want to trip and fall flat on my face in front of thousands of people. After the photographer took my picture, I turned to look for my parents in the crowd; all I could see was a fuzzy sea of wavy colors.

That night we celebrated in typical Nordyke fashion: lots of food, lots of gifts, and lots of laugher with those we love. As the party died down, I felt a compelling need to move on as well—to start on the next phase of my life. As cliché as it sounds, graduation was not an end, it was truly a beginning. I still had dreams, three dreams, to chase, and at least one of them appeared to be on the horizon. Before graduation from Seminole Community College, a very blond young man had been making his way between classes when he heard a voice, an echo of a voice he hadn't heard in more than ten years. The voice said, "I need to get a coke. My blood sugar is low." *That has to be Linda Nordyke!* he thought. He searched the Student Center trying to find me but my voice was carried away in the crowd and he had to get to his class.

God doesn't ask us to give till it hurts—
He simply asks us to give it all.

~ Bill Milliken

The
Greatest
of These

7

*T*HE BLOND BOY HAD GRADUATED FROM HIGH SCHOOL and then attended The University of the South in Sewanee, Tennessee, where his parents financed two years of research in fraternity life. His grades reflected his success in that endeavor, and he found himself making a gentleman's agreement with the University's academic dean: Leave the school, get his act together, and then re-apply for admission to Sewanee after proving his academic worth someplace else. Someplace else turned out to be Seminole Community College, Lake Mary, Florida, in the fall of 1985.

After hearing my voice in the Student Center, Greg went home and flipped through the phone book. Although both of our families had moved, we lived in adjacent communities, just a stone's throw from each other again. *Ring, ring,* "This is Greg Hambleton. Is Linda available?" My dad took the call that night. I was babysitting and would not return home until after

11:30 pm. When Dad gave me the message I could barely breathe, let alone think straight.

Quickly, my brain tried to unscramble ten years of silence. *Greg Hambleton? As in toe-headed, hand-holding, kissing-on-the-curb, exchanging-erasers-and-rings . . . that Greg Hambleton?* I found the courage to call him back. The voice on the other end assured me that he was one and the same. This time, however, it was the voice of a man. We talked for three and a half hours. In the wee hours of the morning he asked if he could come over sometime and say hello. When the boy-turned-man showed up on the doorstep, his eyes were vivid blue, his hair was still gorgeous blond. Moving with a confidence that was devoid of cockiness, he treated my parents with polite respect. He stood tall, calm, and collected. Inside the man's body, however, was still the kind and caring heart of the ten-year-old boy that I had once loved.

We talked through the afternoon, laughing about the good old days and catching up on what had happened in the meantime. He casually mentioned that he wasn't dating anyone. I told him that I was. Malcolm was still in the picture at that point. Greg understood and wished me well. And that was that. We didn't see each other throughout the next semester and we didn't try. Greg excelled in his classes, reapplied to The University of the South and moved back to Tennessee where he continued to excel. At the two-year point of our relationship, both Malcolm and I realized that our romance was not going to last, even though our friendship might. Besides, he wasn't nearly as blond as Greg.

In December of '87, I was back in the hospital. Not that that was strange or anything, I had been hospitalized for ketoacidosis so many times that going to the ER was kind of like going to the gas station for an oil change and a fresh tank of gas— pretty much the same thing over and over and over. One afternoon, though, the routine was interrupted when I woke up after a really deep nap—the kind where your mouth hangs open and all the weird sounds come out. Greg was standing in the doorway of my hospital room staring at me. Embarrassed and wondering how long he had been there, I quickly checked to make sure I hadn't drooled all over myself and my pillow.

"Don't worry," he said, "you look beautiful."

We caught up on the previous eighteen months and then commandeered a wheelchair. Greg pushed me outside for my first fresh air in over a week. It was an absolutely gorgeous day in every respect. We started talking, and talking, and talking. Greg didn't even pretend to be sorry that Malcolm was out of the picture, and I wanted so badly to tell Greg how thrilled I was that he might be back in it.

As Greg prepared to leave, my heart began to wrestle with that great question faced by every woman hanging on the precipice of love: *Is he going to kiss me or not!?* He did. Gently, cautiously yet confidently, not presumptuously, but invitingly.

He turned and walked toward the elevators, but I didn't want to leave his invitation unanswered. I scurried from my room, came up behind him, threw my arms around him and said, "I don't want you to leave." Leaving was only temporary, Greg assured me. We would definitely be keeping in touch.

Greg's parents weren't thrilled about his long-distance phone bill that final semester of his senior year. (At least it was far cheaper than his party bills had been during his freshman and sophomore years!) After graduating he came home. In the bliss of early summer we were nearly inseparable, going to movies, the beach, and our favorite restaurants. One day Greg took me down to the Gulf to spend the day at his family's beach house. Gray and overcast skies mixed with the blues of the salty waters; absolutely beautiful. We had a long walk along the beach—talking, hugging and kissing as the waves lapped at our feet. Back at the beach house Greg got down on one knee. I temporarily forgot to breathe.

Greg had gone to a university that was steeped in tradition—where gentlemanly values were still important and esteemed. One tradition was pinning. The men of his fraternity received a badge when they became active members—a very important symbol of lifelong commitment to new brothers. He asked me if I would give him the honor of wearing his fraternity badge as a symbol of our future engagement. I cried. He pinned the badge right over my heart.

I knew what this meant and I could hardly believe it: We were pre-engaged, a ring would be coming, and then one of my lifetime dreams would become a reality. The afternoon exploded into a rush of conversation. The door to the future opened and we would walk through it together! It wouldn't be just me; now everything would be *we*. We talked about kids, we talked about homes, we talked about places we wanted to travel. It was about our life together now. We were swept along in a flood of conversation and dreams, talking excitedly and incessantly.

Greg planned the day perfectly, of course: the beach, the beach house, stops at a couple of really great restaurants. On the way home we rode in silence, just holding each other's hand, soaking it all in for several hours—not an uncomfortable silence, a very *knowing* type of silence. We *knew* where we were going; we knew how we were going to get there. It was the perfect day, and I was positive that I couldn't love him any more than I did at that moment.

When love is in its infancy, the heart is able to filter out what it wishes. Somehow the mind is able to conform reality to the desires of the heart. In our minds everything was wonderful, and it was. He was going off to a great job in Atlanta that promised a great deal of money. He had a good social base there, and I began to imagine starting a new life with him as soon as possible.

In his mind, Greg also knew that I had diabetes. He wasn't ignorant; it's just that he didn't *really* know. Knowing comes from hearing and seeing. Up to this point, Greg had only seen me go into a low blood sugar situation once (and that was quickly remedied with the help of my mom at our house). Other than that, he didn't truly know what he was getting into (and really, neither did I).

Back in Atlanta, as Greg resumed his carefree bachelor life, his friends began bringing up the issue of my diabetes. *Are you crazy? Do you know what life will be like with a diabetic woman? Are you sure you want to give up everything?* Greg had studied at Oxford for a time, and a friend there and his fiancée took him out to dinner. The fiancée had some medical background and started spelling out the types of things Greg could anticipate. As a twenty-two-year-old bachelor, he began to *really* think about these things. That evening he did his best to take a future inventory of what life would be like with me. The promise of hardship from a chronic degenerative disease meant he would have to sacrifice many facets of life that he held very dear. Greg's family, for example, traveled extensively, including trips overseas. Understandably he didn't want to stop doing that. He questioned whether he had the will to find a way. Back in his apartment he wrote me an eight-page letter.

In our family, it is now known as *The* Letter. But you have to pronounce it properly. It is not "the letter," it is *Theeee* Letter. We gave him high marks for honesty and foresight, but the worst part was that every paragraph or so he repeated a phrase in big bold capitals, underlined and with an exclamation point: BUT REMEMBER, I LOVE YOU!

I read the letter to my family at the dinner table and I narrated it beautifully. I played the part, reading it with exaggerated passion, particularly the line that repeatedly said, "But remember, I loooooove you!" Only I added a little expletive of my own after each of those phrases. I called him all sorts of things. My family laughed and jeered as I mocked him. We were softening the blows, as we normally do, with humor. But it was just a defensive tactic. Everyone knew that I was hurt. Really hurt.

> The door to the future opened and we would walk through it together! It wouldn't be just me; now everything would be *we*.

Yet another kind of pain.

Greg thought he could love me in spite of my disease. He wanted to separate me from diabetes, as if it were an option on a new car he was buying, as if I somehow had the choice of getting rid of it. Maybe he felt like he could love just the part of me that was healthy. But I was a package deal: *If you get me, you get the diabetes, too.* No options. The realization hit me, too: *I'm not this disease, but it's as much a part of me as anything else.* By rejecting the diabetes, he was, therefore, rejecting me, too.

Ouch. *Big ouch.* My heart was so far down the road with

him—our plans, our dreams—now my heart was ripped out. I wanted to be angry and not feel anything for him, but I just couldn't. I was mad at myself and I was mad at him—and yet I still loved him very much. It was a horrible quandary to be in. A phone conversation (ironically on Valentine's Day), was the nail in the coffin. He reiterated to me that even though he cared for me deeply, he couldn't deal with giving up everything to be married to a diabetic. I was going to be his proverbial ball and chain and he cherished his freedom.

"I care for you deeply," Greg said.

"Greg, caring and loving are totally different things, and if you're just caring, let's say goodnight."

And that's what we did. We said goodnight.

Two days later the Cadillac smashed into my car in front of the convenience store. (Not a great week.)

Love.

The musician sings about it. The poet writes about it. The movies try to portray it. The apostle Paul wrote:

> Faith, hope and love abide, but the greatest of these three is love. (1 Corinthians 13:13)

The New Testament was written in Greek, and the Greeks have at least three different words for love. The first, philia, refers to the heartfelt love of friendship (captured in the beer drinking, backslapping buddy's proclamation, "I love you, man!"). The second kind of love, eros, is physical and erotic (the kind of love that can be made in the backseat of a car between two strangers). And finally, there is *agape* love—a supernatural love that loves for the sake of love itself . . . a love that is blind to shortcomings, impervious to imperfection and forgives sin. I have no question in my mind that Greg and I shared the first two kinds of love. Our friendship was deep. As far as the physical stuff goes, the chemistry was definitely there (even though we were committed to stay out of the laboratory until we had rings on).

Greg was standing at the edge of unconditional, agape love. And he had wisely realized that he was unwilling to take the step to live it out. He liiiiiiiiiiiiiiked me, but he didn't loooooooooove me. My parents, sympathetic as usual, said I should be thankful that he had figured this out now rather than later. I supposed they were right.

I emphatically told everyone not to tell Greg about the car accident. I didn't want him running back to me in sympathy like I was some sort of charity case in the midst of a tragedy. No, if he really looooooooooved me, he would have to come back on his own volition. And if he didn't, he was still going to have to come back. I had kept his fraternity badge. If he wanted to pin it on someone else, he was going to have to look me in the eye and explain why she was better than I was.

Greg re-immersed himself in his solo single social life back in Atlanta. A year and a half ticked away while I simmered in the back of his mind and heart. Having ping-ponged from Georgia to Tennessee and then Tennessee to Florida, Greg was now living and working in Miami. During the holidays, he threw a Christmas party for his co-workers. A cup or two of punch later, he started telling them our story. By the time he was done everyone was crying. They said, "What are you doing? You are in love with this woman! Are you a fool? Why in the world don't you marry her?"

Greg came back to Orlando for New Year's, and four or five more cups of punch got him thinking about me again. We were away in St. Louis enjoying our traditional Christmas celebration, but he called the house and left a message on the machine: Ten minutes of slurred babble about how much he wished I was in town and how much he missed me. He woke up the next day and thought, *Oh God, what have I done? What will these people think of me now?* My parents, quite wisely, erased the message and never told me about it—even though Greg had said he still loooooved me.

Another year and a half passed. I was moving on with life, too. But in the back of my mind and heart Greg was always there. Outwardly I was moving on, but inside I was still waiting. I thought maybe Greg just needed a little more time to grow up—time to reassess the good things about me against the realities of diabetes. But after three years of no contact, I had waited about as long as I could. Under the guise of just wanting to wish him happy birthday, I called his former workplace in Tennessee. "He's moved back to Florida," they said. *Oh my God, he's close. He could be here. Maybe close enough to kiss.* I called his parents and asked if they wouldn't mind passing on the message that I had called. I was just wishing him happy birthday, right?

The message was relayed to Miami where Greg was dating another girl. She was probably every man's dream and epitomized everything Greg thought he wanted. Her family was very wealthy. They had a huge home south of Miami in a private enclave with sailboats and yachts and cars galore. They lived life on the cocktail circuit, moving from party to party. When she and her family went to travel through Europe for a couple of months, they left Greg to watch their gorgeous home, and to think. Finally, everything that he thought he wanted was right in front of him, but the dream had lost its luster. Up close the sparkle was superficial and what seemed to promise so much fullness felt empty. It was the perfect time to get a message from me.

Greg called back. Cautiously we began to talk, then we talked a little more, and then we talked, and talked, and talked. My dad kept coming into my room saying, "Are you done yet? Are you done yet?" The last time he came in, it was 2:15 in the morning; he just threw his hands up and said, "Whatever."

When we hung up, Greg realized that he'd experienced more with me in a four hour phone call than he had in his six-month relationship with his girlfriend. When she came back from Europe and returned to college, the breakup was short and to the point, both of them ready to move on. When he came up to Orlando to see me, embers fanned back into flame. We stood again on the edge of pursuing a different kind of love. First, however, Greg had to take a deep gulp and show his face at the Nordyke house—his first time with my family since *The* Letter. Let's say everyone was cordial, except Karen, of course. She was still mad and ready to protect me. She acknowledged his presence but stared at him with one eyebrow raised the whole time.

Greg survived the cool reception but was eager to get out of the house. We went to a movie (neither of us remember which one, but we held hands as we walked out of the theater). Greg looked down at me and said, "Linda, I love you. I have never not loved you. I'm a fool for having broken up with you." I didn't give him the pleasure of crying. I just smiled and said, "I know."

Greg just about wore out his car driving from Miami to Orlando and back every weekend. By March of 1992, he was ready to ask for my hand and knew it was time for him to have "the talk" with my parents. I nervously went to some friends' house for a huge and fun-filled dinner party while Greg went to my house to meet with Mom and Dad.

It was not a done deal.

My dad started by saying, "Greg, when Linda's sister got engaged, all we had to say to them was 'Congratulations. Have a great life.' You obviously had your concerns several years ago about marrying my daughter. Everything that you were concerned about still exists. We need to talk about that." And talk they did—Greg refers to it as a two-hour verbal odyssey. While I bit my nails at the dinner party, my parents let Greg have it all. They went into great detail about every facet of life that was going to be difficult, emotionally trying, and financially demanding. They went into details about the probability of losing limbs, strokes, heart attacks. Greg nodded his head and listened intently. But inside he thought, *It can't be that bad. Look at Linda. She looks great. There's no way it's going to be that bad. It's going to be great for us.*

As the hours ticked away, I became increasingly nervous. I wasn't afraid that mom and dad would say "no." They knew that I was in love with him. It wasn't about whether they would give permission; it was whether or not they would talk Greg out of it. We had been down this road before. *After he has again*

He wanted to separate me from diabetes, as if it were an option on a new car he was buying, as if I somehow had the choice of getting rid of it. Maybe he felt like he could love just the part of me that was healthy.

weighed all the baggage that I was bringing with me, will he still want me? After an eternity, Greg showed up at the party. "We're good to go," he said with a smile.

Greg decided to wait to stage an official engagement. I knew it was coming, but when? We still went out a lot, but he just wouldn't make the move. One night he even took me out to a great dinner. It was killing me; driving me nuts. *Is he ever going to ask?* Not during drinks, or dinner, or dessert, or coffee . . . . *What is he waiting for?* The opportunity passed. *More waiting? What's his problem?!* After dinner we strolled leisurely down Park Avenue. The Winter Park Arts Festival was in full swing. We wandered aimlessly down the Avenue looking in shop windows. A large group had congregated in front of one window and we went up to see what was going on. My eyes took a few moments to focus on what was causing all the interest. When they did, tears welled up in them. The crowd started cheering and, clapping as Greg reached into his pocket and pulled out my ring.

In the window hung a huge sign, *"My Dearest Linda . . . . Will You Marry Me?"*

I was crying so hard that I forgot to say "Yes." We kissed and the crowd clapped louder . . . . The perfect night; perfect. That was March 20, 1992. Seventeen years earlier, to the day, I had asked Greg to be my boyfriend back in elementary school. I didn't think I could possibly love him any more than I did that night.

With the ring on my finger, time started moving again. We had been in love for so long that time had seemed to stand still.

Now, everything was in the future. We had our whole lives to look forward to. Nearly immediately, though, medical issues began to show their face. Greg moved back to Orlando and was ready to take a promising job with a growing company . . . but their insurance benefits were incredibly expensive. Greg had accumulated a tremendous amount of credit card debt buying me gifts and taking me out to expensive dinners. We had to postpone the wedding, knowing that there wasn't enough money waiting on the other side. It was time to seriously tighten the belt, downsize, and cut back.

The financial struggles, however, were nothing compared to what we faced shortly after Thanksgiving.

Dr. Crocket had made good on a promise. So many years before, I had asked him to keep me alive until I lived out my dreams of finding true love, being a mother of my own child, and living a disease-free life. Over the months he had watched with a smile as Greg and I moved toward the altar. But it was a bittersweet smile. He knew that the realization of one dream would mean the loss of another.

In his office, his kind words were mixed with tears and matter-of-fact professionalism. Greg and I sat listening. Dr. Crocket's words were simple enough; they just seemed so surreal in light of the bliss that we had been experiencing in the former months. He talked about my seizures, about the affects of swings in my blood sugar, about the devastating stress that would be placed on my body. The bottom line was simply this:

If I were to become pregnant, both my life and that of our child could be in jeopardy.

Together we talked about all possibilities and options, about the developmental issues that our baby would face, and about specific risks to my health. We thought through each option, and each one led to an unacceptable dead end. Planned pregnancy was out of the question. An unplanned pregnancy would be equally devastating, probably forcing the decision to have a therapeutic abortion (a scenario that I could not endure).

The final conclusion was as brutal as it was obvious. A flood of emotion and thought followed the familiar course all must travel when dreams die: *denial, bargaining, anger, depression,* and—at the bottom of an ocean of tears—*acceptance.*

I had to walk through it all again. A fresh diagnosis with fresh and painful repercussions. I should have seen it coming, really. Childlessness is so common for those with my disease. But the dream was so vivid that I was blindsided. *A forever-empty womb; a forever-empty corner of my heart.* To make matters worse, as I walked through the process of absorbing the news, I felt like I was alone. This was the first major medical issue that Greg and I faced together and Greg took it very well. *Too well,* I thought. His cool indifference to a future of childlessness left me feeling alone with the death of my dream and the grief and mourning for things that would never be. I turned to my dad for consolation; he is the more outwardly emotional one, and together we cried buckets of tears. But Greg and my mom? They were a different story. At first I felt like they didn't care, but that's not true at all. Both of them are just very practical in a crisis, very matter-of-fact, almost clinical about things that I find very emotional. I resented that at the time, but in the years since I've come to see that too is a gift—part of the balance of the team of people with which God surrounded me.

Neither mom nor Greg gets upset very often. They seem to know their energy is better used somewhere else, where they can help, when they need to be strong for those of us who, like my dad and me, often succumb to emotions.

In the end, it really didn't matter who was feeling what. On December 8, 1992, with a cut of the scalpel, the dream of having a child of my own was severed.

That Christmas was a real mixture of thankfulness and wrestling with the "why" question. The man of my prayers and dreams held me in his arms, but I knew that I would never have children of my own to hold in mine. My branch of the family tree would grow no further.

As if to add insult to injury, God gave me a daily reminder of my barrenness several years later when I awoke from a nap with a wet shirt. It was breast milk. I immediately thought *breast cancer*. A CAT scan of the brain, however, revealed a tumor. *A brain tumor? Please dear God, please dear God, please dear God.* My mind raced into the fear of the worst, but Dr. Crocket said, "No, just wait. Sometimes tumors form in the brain on the pituitary gland; it's called a prolactinoma. You're going to be fine. We'll just have to keep an eye on it and every now and then check the size to make sure it's okay. It does seem, if you're going to be lactating for awhile, you'll need to buy some bra pads that nursing mothers wear."

The fear of cancer was softened by Dr. Crockett's words, but it was quickly replaced by an emotional sting. I was lactating, producing milk for a baby that I didn't have and wouldn't have. Again, none of this seemed to make sense. There are plenty of mothers who have trouble lactating; there are plenty of mothers who don't want to be mothers. I wanted to be a mother and I couldn't. Now I was getting a daily reminder of my childlessness.

It was another closet moment, a handful of critical minutes when honesty overflowed into anger before God. Why would God give me such an incredible desire for something, deny me, and then rub it in my face? I had nurtured the dream of being a mother for so long, the innate drive to love a child was overwhelming. I still wonder with whom I am supposed to share this one-of-a-kind love. If it's not meant to be my child, who? I haven't come up with anybody yet.

> There are physical limits to the human condition, and these limits have little respect for our dreams.

After I cut loose on God yet again, I somewhat apologized for what I said. *Please forgive me, but You've got to understand how I feel.* As He has so many times, God and His peace met me there, again, offering no real answers to my questions, but replacing the anger with a joy that reached beyond my loss. Tim Hansel described it this way:

> *But there is no such thing as cheap joy. Joy often costs pain and suffering. True joy isn't at the end of a rainbow. It isn't captured at the top of the ladder of success. Its price tag is faithfulness, endurance, and perhaps sorrow. It has been suggested that our cup of joy can only be as deep as our cup of sorrow.*[23]

The lactation lasted for four years and four months—a damp, soggy reminder of my empty womb. Why so long? Was there some lesson I was supposed to learn? I was in this class-room daily and I think I handled it pretty well. I was ready to move on, but just because we pass some sort of exam doesn't mean we graduate from hardship. Go through it, whether you learn from it or not.

My mom had actually offered to carry a child for Greg and me. We considered that, as well as adoption. But in reality, there wasn't a judge anywhere that would give us a child with my medical history. The sicker I became, the more obvious it became that bringing a child into our family wasn't going to work. There are physical limits to the human condition, and these limits have little respect for our dreams.

Finding joy in the suffering seems to be the continual challenge, at least it was for us. Financial struggles continued and my parents strongly suggested a second time that we postpone the wedding. They may have been expecting another letter like *The* Letter to show up shortly. But it never did. We worked things out; we talked them through. Greg continued to show a side of himself that melted the hearts of my family and confirmed what I already deeply knew to be true about him. Before we even had a chance to make it down the aisle, the agape love of God was trickling into our lives. Superhuman sacrifice and dedication was moving though his life to mine. This was the man for me, and I was the one for him.

I wish I could go back and pay more attention. I wish I could go back and replay it all in moment-by-moment snap shots. I wish I could go back and savor every second, every smell, every sound, every word. Once just wasn't enough, particularly since all of it was blurred by tears of gratefulness. I was simply overwhelmed by the fact that it was happening, that I had lived long enough to get married.

Friends and family came from all corners of the country. Dr. Crocket was there, as was Grandpa. Grandma wasn't—not in person at least, but I believe that she looked down in spirit as I wore her diamond jewelry and carried her favorite embroidered handkerchief. As the formalities began, Aunt Peggie, Uncle John, and my cousin Judy presented the most resonating rendition of John Denver's song "Perhaps Love" that I had ever heard. The words described love as a shelter when it storms, a window through which new vistas can be seen, a door through which lovers walk toward the future together. Love is comforting, protecting, inviting, though sometimes painful, and sometimes full of fire or thunder, as two become one and their dreams come true, as mine were coming true for me at that very moment!

I peeked between the doors as everyone took their places. At the front stood the blond boy, the one and only human with whom I knew I could spend my life. God had chosen him; He had chosen us for each other; and somehow He had preserved us through the decades leading to this day. There was the long slow walk to the altar, loved ones lined up at our left and our right. "Who then, gives this woman to this man?" "Her mother and I do," said my dad, as he took my hand and placed it in Greg's. The chime of the bell choir reverberated, the candles flickered, the pastor prayed. Simple formalities, echoing through the generations, as we became a family of our own, now responsible for each other, dependent on each other. With my hand in Greg's hand, I entrusted him with my heart and my life, quite literally.

For better or for worse, in sickness or in health, for richer or for poorer, till death do us part.

Few couples that walk down the aisle, caught up in the pomp and celebration, deeply understand the true implication of those words. With attraction and passion pumping through the veins at light speed, could any of us have imagined that agape love would be so different and cost so much? Greg made a commitment, a conscious choice of his will, but could he have known what lay ahead?

No, not that day. No matter how long my parents talked to him, no matter how much he studied about my disease, how could he have known? How can *anyone* know when they make that vow what really waits down the road? How could we ever have known the struggles and difficulties that would push us past the edge of our physical and emotional resources, forcing us to redefine love in our own hearts?

Broken expectations and broken bodies are strewn like litter on the road to true agape love. And along the way comes the tragic discovery that we don't, in and of ourselves, have the capacity to love in such a way. Our human nature includes too much selfishness, too much regret, too much exhaustion. Completing the journey requires a choice, and another choice, and then another choice. Each of us must choose to dip into another source of love—love from the One who touched the leper, the One who is the friend of the prostitute—and then let that love from God Himself flow to those around us.

It is a surrender of sorts, an admission, "I can't love like this, Lord," followed by the sincere plea " . . . but please love through me." I believe that God answers such prayers. In fact, I believe pain and difficulty may have been designed by God to generate an ongoing dependency on Him, leading to an ongoing intimacy with Him as our Creator, our Lord, and the Lover of our souls as we seek to love those around us. For when we need to love the most, and when we seem to be able to give it the least, doesn't it make sense that it's God calling us to Himself? Could all this be an invitation from Him to work through us, so that He can become our sufficiency and become the love that others need so desperately?

We stood at the altar where we left our past behind and stepped across the threshold into a grand adventure into a new kind of love. *For better or for worse, in sickness or in health, for richer or for poorer, till death do us part.* I didn't think I could ever love him more than I did that day.

But I was wrong.

Just as each of us has a unique fingerprint, so each of us has a unique inner personal gift. We are all the poorer if we do not encourage it to be released in others, nor release our own.

~ Robert Raines

You can survive on your own. You can grow strong on your own. You can even prevail on your own. But you cannot become human on your own.

~ Frederick Buechner

Blood Relatives

8

*I*T WAS APRIL 15, 1997. TAX DAY. (We should know better than to get out of bed on that day.) I say we petition to have that day removed from the calendar all together. Just kind of skip it, pretend that it didn't happen. For the months prior to that day, I was floating on Cloud 9 with no ground in sight. Newly wed and feeling great, we had the whole world at our fingertips and every star within our reach. But the day taxes were due, I was in the apartment when all of a sudden it felt like Midnight, our cat, had brushed up against my leg. But she didn't. Just a weird sensation, and then my leg suddenly gave out and my whole left side briefly went numb. *Strange, but not a big deal. Look, girl, you're fine again.* I called my parents and Dr. Crockett, but I didn't tell Greg. At least not yet. (Nothing is completely real until I tell Greg, and I guess I didn't want this to be real.) My parents took me to the ER at Florida Hospital Orlando campus.

Later I explained to Greg about TIAs, Transient Ischemic Attacks, which are basically little mini strokes common to diabetics. I tried to downplay it, but complications weren't far behind. I was on very high doses of an anti-seizure medication.

> ". . . if you had to make a choice between losing your ability to speak and losing your sight, which would you choose?"

Sure, it kept me from seizing up, but it also turned me into a wet noodle. At dinner that night, I did a full-on face-plant right into my macaroni and cheese. Greg was looking at his gooey new bride trying to figure out what to do when nature called. So here's Greg, thinking, *Okay how do I do this? She's going to fall into her food; I'm going to pee my pants.* So he took off his necktie, wrapped it around my chest and tied me to the dining room chair. It worked pretty well, actually. He left me tied up for the rest of the meal. We laugh about it now, but at the time it was a frightening realization for Greg:

I was scared and I'm sure Linda was scared because I couldn't imagine that my level of care was anything like she had received from her parents. We had to sleep on a fold-out couch on the main floor because Linda couldn't make the stairs. One night her blood sugar went low. I jumped out of bed at two o'clock in the morning to get her a coke and stubbed my toe on that hideous fold-out bed. When Linda has low blood sugar, she doesn't respond normally; she's much more emotional and volatile. She also gets very hot. I tried to remove her nightgown to help her cool off. She got very embarrassed and started to cry. She thought I was mad at her, but really, I was just mad at the whole scenario. Reality was finally showing its face and I had to begin dealing with real broken expectations—and human nature being what it is, I felt a lot of fear, anger, sadness, and disillusionment. When you're stressed a lot of things come out.

Some of our struggles were just typical adjustments for newlyweds, but with diabetes in the picture all the issues got turned up to high and started to boil over. I felt exposed, like I had no protection, and I didn't, not for my body and not for my soul. I felt very vulnerable and very defensive. I was sick all the time. Greg would come home from work and would have to take care of me from the moment he walked through the door. When things started to really get tough, Greg finally took me to the hospital. That was a real wake-up call for us. Soon enough though, I stabilized and we were able to put it behind us. *Nothing to get distracted with*, I told myself. Besides, I didn't want anyone telling me that I needed to stop or slow down. We went back to living the dream and soon got back on track. My body cooperated with good feelings and great looks, and I was in love with the blonde boy more than I could ever possibly imagine. We were also working ourselves out of financial debt. I had a great new job and my career was on the fast track. I was sprinting through training, jumping over promotions and pacing myself for upper management. Just before New Year's Eve we bought a piece of land and began building our dream home. It was all just really, really good.

I was living fast and furiously. Sure, there were little things that hurt, twinges that seemed a little bit out of whack, but I was too busy enjoying life to pay attention. Greg, not knowing what I should have been doing, asked now and then if we shouldn't see a doctor. "I've got it all taken care of; everything is fine," I told him. But in fact I wasn't even testing my blood sugars as I should have been. (I usually ran my blood sugar four to six times a day; now I was lucky to squeak out that many in two to three days.)

I took the mind-over-matter approach; I was sure that a positive mental attitude would triumph over physical challenges. I thought that if I didn't accept it, it wasn't real. I know better now. I know that in order to exercise the power of mind-over-matter, you have to know what is the matter and *then* put your mind to it. I now know that when you have a real problem, that problem is real, whether you accept it or not. I didn't do that. Throughout 1999 I had been living in denial, ignoring clear warning signs and symptoms. I pretended all was well, but in reality, I was going deeper and deeper into ESRD—End Stage Renal Disease. My kidneys were ready to fail.

The sun went down on February 15, 2000, just as blissfully as it had for the last three years. The dawn of February 16 was another story. Greg was up and getting ready for work. My head was killing me; I asked him to go downstairs and make some coffee. I had one of those awkward nauseous feelings, but I didn't really chalk it up to anything. *Headaches are the norm for so many of us, right?* When he came back up he found me lying half paralyzed on the bed.

"Linda's whole right side had just dropped. She was hanging

off the bed like a rag doll. She was trying to speak, but the sounds were coming out in unintelligible gurgles and slurs," Greg says. He dialed 911 and then stayed on the line until he could hear the sirens of the paramedics approaching the apartment.

"Aaaaay uuuunt issssstik. Aaaaay uuuunt issssstik." A new sense of aloneness pierced my soul. I had clear thoughts in my mind; an important message formulated in my head, but I couldn't get it out.

Greg came close to listen more carefully, "What? What is it?"

"Aaaaay uuuunt issssstik!" I was a prisoner in my own brain trying desperately to connect with my loved one only a few inches away. No matter how urgently I tried, I was alone with my thoughts.

"Aaaaay uuuunt issssstik!"

"You want . . . what?"

"Issssstik!"

Greg crinkled his forehead. "You want . . . . lipstick?"

Within a few minutes of the paramedics' arrival, I could begin to force out the words that seemed stuck inside my head, although they still came out blurred and distorted. At the stroke unit of Florida Hospital, called the SMART Unit, Dr. Crockett came in and read me the riot act. He just chewed me out—up one side and down the other. "Linda! Where have you been for the last year and a half? What have you been doing?" He let Greg have it, too. "You know what to do! This is so important to

> I was more afraid now that I *wouldn't* die, that I would have to live with this worse than excruciating pain.

keep in check! This is a job for both of you!" I was scared this time more than the last, for sure, but still pretty sure that everyone was just being overly protective.

Greg brought me pretzels, which I was munching enthusiastically when the weirdest thing happened: I was lying in my hospital bed strapped down by at least 101 wires and cables and tubes, holding a pretzel in my hand, when it disappeared—not just the pretzel, but my hand, too. I was looking at both the hand and the pretzel, but I couldn't tell they were there; it was a total disconnect between my body and my brain. Then my hand that wasn't there dropped limp to my side, and then my whole right side went limp. My eyes drooped, the corner my mouth went slack and drool dribbled to my chin. Total rag doll.

Greg screamed for the nurse; other nurses rushed in, checked my vitals, tried to get me to move, and asked me questions. Again, the sentences formed in my head, but no one could understand a word I was saying. I was imprisoned in my mind once again, and this time I believed I was in trouble, real, tangible, wake-up-and-smell-the-

> Most women look at food and the only thing they have to ask is, "Is it going to make me fat?" I had to look at food and say, "Is this going to kill me?"

coffee trouble. I started to cry. *Will I be stuck in here, alone, forever?* Instinctively I wanted to pray, but I had no idea of what to ask for at first, but then it was obvious. *Please don't let me die.* And then, *Please don't let this be permanent. Not alone forever.*

A brain angiogram revealed a blood clot. It appeared to be huge. They strapped me to a gurney and rushed toward surgery. I kept telling them that I was feeling sick. But they said "Oh no, no. We've given you something for the nausea. You're fine. You're fine. You're fine." I wasn't fine and I knew it. Dr. Frank Huang-Hellinger finally looked at me and said, "Flip her over!" So they turned me over and I barfed all over the floor and his shoes. "Can't say she didn't warn me," Dr. Hellinger said. We all laughed, but the laugher wasn't sustained.

Dr. Hellinger softened none of his words. This was a matter of life and death. He told me that even if I were to survive the procedure, I could lose my sight, or the ability to speak. "I don't think you're going to die, but that is a real possibility. You need to know that," he said. "But I need to know something, because once I'm in there, I may have to make some choices. Linda, if you had to make a choice between losing your ability to speak and losing your sight, which would you choose?"

A long pause. *This is not some random job interview question. This is not a youth group icebreaker. This is not hypothetical. This is real.*

A wind of seriousness blew through my soul. *This is real; this is real. Think, think.* I had survived the darkness. I had been there before and learned to thrive; but a lifetime of keeping my mouth shut? That seemed incomprehensible. "If you have to choose," I said, "take my eyes." And with that they put the mask over my face and I slipped into the darkness, wondering if I would ever see light again.

With great relief, the clot was not as large as anticipated. When anesthesia wore off, I opened my eyes and a flood of light rushed toward my brain. My mouth worked, too. God had spared me one more time. My denial over the last several years, however, would have immediate and long-term consequences. I had started a domino effect, triggering a string of medical problems that began to tumble out of control.

On April 5 of that year, Dr. Joel D. Greenberg did a heart catheter to check my arteries. But the amount of dye that he had to use tipped me over into complete kidney failure. I also experienced a second myocardial infarction—not a massive heart attack, but a heart attack nonetheless. One of the results was yet another kind of pain that rushed through my body—my *whole* body. It hurt to breathe; it hurt to move. If I moved my leg an inch I almost wanted to die; in fact, I thought I was dying. I had no idea what was wrong with me, but I was scared. How could I hurt this much and not be dying? I was certain that I was dying and they just didn't have the guts to tell me. This was the first time I realized that my kidneys were more than just threatened, they were clearly terminal. I had been given warnings—the swelling in my legs on business trips for example—but I overlooked them. My last thought at that particular moment was simple: I was more afraid now that I *wouldn't* die, that I would have to live with this worse than excruciating pain.

Sometimes I wish I could play the tape over again. If only I had gone to see Dr. Crockett earlier. If only I had been honest about the signs and symptoms. *If only, If only, If only* . . . . I had been too busy living the life that I always wanted. I ignored reality for a lot of reasons: feeling foolish, money, not wanting to impose. I suppose it was denial more than anything. The simple questions of an informed physician would have yielded answers that I didn't want to face.

None of us knew how delicate my kidneys were until it was too late. At that point it was just too late. In April I was informed that I would probably need a kidney transplant within three to five years. In July I was told that three to five years was reduced to *now*. I needed the kidney ASAP. But there is no such thing as a kidney store. It requires a donor, someone who is willing to part with one of two kidneys. The surgery for a donor is extensive, and left with one kidney, the person must consider the prospects should something go wrong with the remaining one.

Still, the search did not take long. My mom said she always knew that she was going to be the one, even before there was a need. She knew her blood type was O positive, but we didn't know what mine was. We later discover it, too, was O positive. Without hesitation the woman who gave me life knew she would do so one more time. She wasn't the only one to step forward. My maternal aunt and uncle also got in line without hesitation, as did both my Aunt Peggie's daughters, Becky and Patti. One of my best friends, James P. Donnelly (also my boss at the time) and several others wanted the opportunity to save me. I'm not sure what to say about that. I was overwhelmed, of course. I still am.

I was shocked by Mom's sacrifice, but I was hardly surprised. That's the way she is. That's the way she's always been. Mom is my *Steel Magnolias*. (If you've seen the movie, you know what I

A matching pancreas had just become available. If we were in the ER by 11:00, it would be mine.

mean.) The movie hit too close to home for comfort, but it did give an accurate dramatic presentation of what many diabetics face. Against doctor's orders, the daughter (played by Julia Roberts) chose to get pregnant and carried her baby to full-term. The pregnancy blew her kidneys and she had to go on dialysis. Her mother (played by Sally Field) gave her one of her kidneys. The ending, however, was different from mine. Again failing to recognize her limitations, the daughter pushed her body beyond its abilities. She ended up on life support and they eventually had to let her go.

The morning of December 6, 2000, Gregory Ellis, a Florida Hospital Chaplain, stood between two gurneys. Holding my mom's hand on one side and my hand on the other, he asked for God's peace and presence, and for skill and wisdom for the physicians who would transfer the life-giving organ from one of us to the other. When he left, my mom and I reached out and held each other's hands, and captured each other's gaze. Profound moments—nothing theoretical, nothing hypothetical. This was real; this was real life and I was saturated in it.

They wheeled my mom away and began to cut her open, preparing to take out her left kidney. They wheeled me away and cut me open, preparing my body to receive it. In the waiting room our family prayed and paced back and forth. In the operating room the complex transfer of life was taking place. When they were done, my new kidney started working immediately. They tell me I peed all over the operating table. That may not mean much to some people, but prior to the transplant my body could process only about 100 cc of urine a day. So peeing on the operating table? That was huge; a really good sign. Mom came out okay, too.

The two of us recovered at my parents' house. We shared the master bed, lying side by side as our insides sloshed around, a very strange feeling. (We had been majorly replumbed, and it would take a while before all the pipes settled down in their new places.) That gave us days to contemplate what we had just been through. We didn't have much to say, yet it was one of the most incredible bonding seasons that I've ever had with my mom or anyone else. (And I doubt that I'll ever experience anything like that again). We've always had a strong soul connection, but now we had just been through this life-changing event together; now we shared a vital organ between us. It was just before Christmas and the festive and joyous celebration of the season made that time together even more magical.

It was almost as though the kidney had a life of its own. We even joined in a strange tradition that is shared by many transplant patients. We gave the kidney a name: Jean, which was my maternal Grandma's first name and my mom's and my middle name. Since these three "Jeans" had a part in making all this happen, that was really the only name to choose. We still celebrate Jean's birthday every December 6th. We exchange gifts and the whole works. On March 27, which is my mom's birthday, she gives Jean a present as well. (Yes, that's strange, I know, but it's a celebration of the miracle—a recognition of the mystery of the gift of life that is shared between us all.)

While we were still recovering, Karen's in-laws prepared a full Christmas dinner for us and brought it down from Daytona Beach. It came in one great big crate; I mean it was huge. They delivered it Christmas morning totally prepared, ready to eat. We have had plenty to celebrate every other Christmas, but that Christmas we touched a different level of awe. I was celebrating a new awareness of life. My mom, who gave me life the first time, had given it to me all over again. The parallels with the Christmas story that we were celebrating did not go unnoticed.

That was 2000. It ended well, but I was very glad to have that year in the rear-view mirror.

Hardship, pain, disease; it's an opportunity, really, a window through which we can see life in new ways; it's a door that invites us into a new passage on this journey. Through it we learn the art of giving. Because of it we may have to learn to receive for the first time—vulnerable, unguarded receiving from others, ourselves, and our God.

"Jean" stayed healthy and she remains that way to this day. Kidneys are so vulnerable to my disease. Once the pancreas goes, the kidney is usually not far behind. Protecting it is a primary concern. That's why Dr. Warren and Dr. Crockett approached me about the idea of another transplant, a pancreas transplant.

My insulin pump was doing a near adequate job of controlling the diabetes, but a truly functioning pancreas that was naturally making my own insulin would obviously be much, much better. The possibility ignited a fresh fire under a distant dream: If I had a new healthy pancreas, my disease would be . . . gone. *I could live my dream of a disease-free life!* Pancreas transplants are relatively new; it wasn't even a possibility when I was younger. *A disease-free life?* I couldn't even imagine it. I mean, I really couldn't. Yes, back there on the edge of my memories I had fuzzy recollections of life without diabetes, but after more than three decades of needles, I just couldn't imag-

> In the midst of the pain, I had just begun to live a miracle, in my dream.

ine not checking my blood sugar, or not calculating how much glucose was in a specific food, or being fearful that I was going to damage my kidney. Most women look at food and the only thing they have to ask is, "Is it going to make me fat?" I had to look at food and say, "Is this going to kill me?"

The possible benefits were huge. But it wasn't without risk. My body had been through so much already and my heart was weak. While my parents thought a successful transplant would be miraculous, Greg had deep concerns, but he fully engaged, trying to find out as much as he could. He came with me on every consultation and he read like crazy. He met with the transplant coordinators, which was important. He needed to know these people to build some trust and so did I. The transplant took place outside of Florida Hospital and that was scary. The way people interacted with us was not what we were used to. We were used to a different level of care and concern. We were nervous at first, but at the same time, we knew they were the ones available on a professional level with my current insurance. It would have been nice to have had both, but in the end we were confident that they had what it would take to do the job well. Greg came on board and we decided to move ahead.

The Bible says that it is more blessed to give than to receive. I don't have any reason to doubt that is true, except that I have been so incredibly blessed as a receiver of other people's giving. Sometimes I wonder if it isn't more difficult to receive than give, however. Several weeks prior to our transplant, my mom and I were in the conference room of Shands Hospital in Gainesville. We struck up a conversation with a woman who needed a kidney transplant. Her daughter was a match and willing to be her donor, but the woman couldn't bring herself to accept it. The sacrificial gift just seemed too much. (This happened around Easter, by the way, and the parallels didn't go unnoticed.)

My mom and I pulled her aside. "She's doing the most wonderful thing you can imagine. She wants you here as long as possible." My mom told the woman to give her daughter what she wanted most; she wanted her mother, and she wanted to give. In order to give the daughter what she wanted, the mother needed to learn to receive—just like me. Through our story the woman's heart changed. It was one of those really cool moments when you know God puts you in the right place at the right time with the right message. We left that day feeling better than we had in a long time. We felt we had been placed there for a purpose.

The process of finding a donor who is a match is rarely speedy. A week passed. Then another. Then another. I kept calling the scheduler and saying, "I haven't heard from you. I was kind of wondering when you might get me on the top of that list." And she would say "Well, Linda there's this thing we call 'protocol'. We have a system of priorities and procedures that must be followed." Boy, I hated all the red tape of "protocol." I thought, *How complicated can this be? You take my name, you write it on the top of the list, and boom, the next pancreas that comes along is mine. You're a big hospital. You've got to have plenty of pancreases lying around; just put me on the top list!* Of course, there is a little more to it than that. For one thing, a donated pancreas comes from a cadaver. I knew that in my head, but I didn't understand it in my heart until March 21, 2003.

At 7:11 that morning, we got the call. A matching pancreas had just become available. If we were in the ER by 11:00, it would be mine. A huge mixture of emotion crashed over us. A tidal wave of excitement and an undertow of fear hit us all at once. Even Mom, who is usually as cool as a cucumber, became unglued and started running around to make last-minute preparations. We rushed to the hospital (just over two hours away in Gainesville, Florida) only to be told to wait, then wait some more. We were anxious and we were frustrated. The unfamiliar faces in an unfamiliar hospital didn't help, neither did our self-centered unawareness of what was happening in other rooms.

While we were waiting, I also did some thinking. I looked at my insulin pump. I looked at the pump again, and then removed the tubes and needles that connected it to my body. I turned off the pump, tossed it in my suitcase and threw the tubes and needles in the garbage. I said, "This is the last time I'm ever going to have anything to do with you!" I was so excited. It was my declaration of independence from disease, the 4th of July was here and it was almost time to set off the fireworks. *That's it, that's the end of it. This is a brand-new life.*

When the time finally came, we shared a lot of prayer, kisses, well-wishing, and hand holding. A flurry of doctors swarmed in. It was now 11 pm on the 21st. The original time for the transplant was supposed to be 1 pm; medicine and organ procurement is tricky business, at best. Nurses introduced themselves.

> It's a strange business, this business of transplants. *Life through death. Giving via receiving.* The possibility of life and health to one family requires the death and despair of another.

The anesthesiologist said hello and then, "Night, night, honey"— the last thing I remember before everything went dark and I was trying to finish another prayer.

When light returned, it came with searing, intense pain. I

had been split open from sternum to pubic bone, leaving a nineteen inch scar where I was literally splayed open. Fifty-nine staples ran up and down, holding me together on the outside. Inside there were many more stitches. The surgery lasted five and a half hours. If any movement of any other part of my body pulled and pushed in that area, it was set on fire. When I could finally talk, I turned to Mom. "Remind me. Why did I do this?" The answer was simple: *Insulin*, a little bio-chemical called *insulin*. And then the news came. My new pancreas was making that little chemical. In the midst of the pain, I had just begun to live a miracle.

Accepting these truths gives us a clear responsibility to live, really live. We have an obligation to thrive and not just survive, to care for our bodies and to be honest about the condition of our souls.

During the hospital recovery, the full story of what had taken place began to soak in. My pancreas transplant had been delayed because someone, a man named Donald, desperately needed a liver transplant. My family got to talking to his family in the waiting room. Through their conversations they made the connection that Donald and I were getting organs from the same donor. Donald's hospital room and mine ended up right next to each other. As soon as we could move, we started visiting each other.

A special bond formed between our families. We are so different in so many ways. He was male, 52, I was 40. He was African-American, I'm Caucasian. But we soon discovered our common faith in Christ, and there was even more to it than that. He began to call me his sister; I begin to call him my brother. Because we shared a relative, we shared blood. My dad, ever the jokester, even began to tease Donald about race issues. "I wonder if you have a white liver or if we have a black pancreas? Or is it the other way around?" Those are things you wouldn't ordinarily laugh about, but those were not ordinary days. The relationship stuck; we still call each other and send birthday cards, anniversary cards, etc. I have been blessed by design, not birth, with a wonderful brother and Bettye, his amazing wife.

There are two sides to every coin. While Donald and I celebrated new life, the cadaver of a nineteen-year-old male was cooling in the basement of the hospital, never to breathe, never to feel the beat of the heart, never to a form a thought again, ever. My pancreas and Donald's liver came to us not through a "protocol," but through a donor, a donor that had a name and a family, a mere boy who just hours before have been living, dreaming, and loving. Through the grapevine we learned that the cadaver's name was Donald as well; however, his grandmother called him Chad. Chad had died in a motorcycle/car accident. He was the only son of two parents, parents who went home to an empty house the same day we celebrated. *New life, purchased by the death and sacrifice of an only son.* I'd heard this story before and the parallels resonated deeply; I was living in a physical illustration of the most important of spiritual truths.

I had been given physical freedom by the death of the only son of a family I never met. I had been given spiritual freedom, forgiveness, and new spiritual life by the only Son of God.

The most precious of gifts are all given without condition through essential and indisputable sacrifices. In God's case, the gift of forgiveness and new life is continually offered. No matter how far we feel we are from Him, no matter how long it takes to recognize His generosity, God never retracts His offer of forgiveness and a new life. But, like the woman whose daughter offered her a kidney, each of us must be willing to receive the gift, to humbly accept the incomprehensibly undeserved gift of kindness.

It's a strange business, this business of transplants. *Life through death. Giving via receiving.* The possibility of life and health to one family requires the death and despair of another. For reasons I'll never know this side of the grave, God immersed me in the wonder of it all. I have a mother who gave me life twice. I have been given a vital organ through the son of parents I will never meet (doesn't that make me their daughter, too?). The Son of God died in my place and then transplanted His life into my heart. Somehow, that makes us all blood relatives. It is stunning and it is real. Through the disease and the pain I've come to accept it all. No more denial for me.

Accepting these truths gives us a clear responsibility to live, really live. We have an obligation to thrive and not just survive, to care for our bodies and to be honest about the condition of our souls.

The reality of disease free-living was even better than I had dreamed. Having insulin without having to give myself a shot—many, many shots—was something that I never thought was going to happen, something that I can only barely remember from those earliest days of childhood. I really didn't have that in my memory. Diabetes had always been my reality. It was incredible. I felt completely free. I wasn't tied to anything. I wasn't tied to an insulin bottle or a pump. No syringes, no shots, no worries when it came time to eat. I could inhale whatever I wanted, when I wanted, and as much as I wanted. It almost became a game. I'd eat ice cream, cookies, cake, and then run my blood sugar just for fun: 87, perfect. Then I'd eat a whole bag of M & Ms and check my blood sugar again: 93, perfect. I mean could that have been any cooler? I don't think so. The fear of harming my kidney evaporated. I had lived with that dark cloud for so long that it was a totally new experience to live in the sunshine without it. The excitement never wore off, though I may have begun to take it for granted a little bit. It was fun; we just cut loose.

I was learning to live all over again. But before I really understood what living meant, I had to learn to die.

I'm not afraid of my death. I just don't want to be there when it happens.

~ Woody Allen

Beyond the
Valley of
the Shadow

9

I COULD SEE A FOG OF DEEP PINK, like a translucent cloud of smoke, flowing in my direction. Moving at will, it pursued me, toyed with me, and poised itself to consume me. Something evil existed in the mist; perhaps the fog itself was evil. It pierced my heart with terror. I ran as fast as I could. As if watching from above, I could see the fog pursuing me and I could see myself utterly alone—a personal horror movie in which I was both the actor and the audience, stalked by something dark, something satanic. To fail to escape would be to succumb to the forces that sought to destroy me, devour me, digest me, kill me. The devil himself was trying to overtake me, coming closer and closer, nipping at my heels.

And then, I would wake up. Disoriented, shaking, horrified, and trying to catch my breath. Every emotion told me that the pink fog was real—a vapor that was hunting me, waiting to take my very soul. Many minutes would pass before I could convince myself that it was just a dream. But in my mind I was never sure. For days, the visions from the nightmare stirred fear and anxiety. Was this demonic? A premonition? A subconscious warning telling me to prepare for something?

I first had that nightmare when I was thirteen. Since then the same images and emotions have invaded my sleep seven times.

> I had asked for a normal life, but I hadn't asked Him for a normal life for *the rest* of my life. Maybe He misunderstood; maybe if I asked again.

Each time the pink fog comes. Each time I try every means of escape. Usually I run. Once I jumped in a car. The last time I ran down a very long dock and fled in a motor boat, or maybe I just thought I was escaping; maybe the fog *let* me get away.

I will probably never know if these dreams were just in my mind or whether they were some sort of reflection of spiritual and physical realities. All I know is that the nightmare gave me an image of something we all know in our head and yet rarely embrace with our hearts: somewhere out there death lurks, waiting for us. Our vulnerability and our mortality is an inescapable mist that is never, never far behind us. In our minds we might think we can outrun it, but that is the only true illusion.

As the old adage goes: The only thing that is for sure is death and taxes.

But as we all know, that's only half true.

Through the early Spring of 2004, I was still relishing a diabetes-free life. By April and May, however, something just didn't seem right. (Granted, it seems like there's always something haywire somewhere in my body, but this was different.) I felt more tired than usual, run down for no reason. My blood sugar levels were still normal. Yet I felt something was amiss. After two years of eating whatever I wanted, I found myself leaving my plate more full than empty. Weird.

In July, lab tests revealed that my amylase and lipase levels were high (these are digestive enzymes and a byproduct made inside the pancreas). The normal numbers for these two enzymes in the body are between 25 and 105; mine were 900 and climbing. It appeared the new pancreas was leaking. Greg and I couldn't believe it. After all I had been through in the past and with all my new freedoms, it just couldn't be true. I felt like I earned that pancreas, that I really deserved it.

The doctors wanted to take a closer look. A CAT scan, comprehensive ultrasound, and two different MRIs revealed nothing. The truth was, they couldn't find the pancreas. It's not uncommon for a pancreas to migrate through the body, but it was disconcerting that it was nowhere to be found. Dr. Timothy Childers, a General Surgeon, was perplexed and concerned about my symptoms. At 10 pm on July 6, 2004, he stood at my bedside telling Greg and me he just didn't know what was going on inside my abdominal cavity, but he would see me at 10:30 am the next day to go in for a look.

At 5:30 the next morning, we were startled awake by the phone. "Mr. and Mrs. Hambleton? I am sorry to get you up so early, but I couldn't sleep for wondering what really is going on in there. I just have to go in for a look around, *now*." Thirty minutes later I was on the operating table prepped for exploratory surgery. Beneath my still new and precious kidney he found what he was looking for: my appendix was completely taken over with gangrene. Dr. Childers could not believe it hadn't ruptured (which probably would have killed me immediately). It was a close call, very close. I had dodged one fatal bullet, and that was a minor miracle. On the other hand, after the whole episode, the tests failed to reveal anything specifically wrong with the pancreas. The doctors were out of ideas. They told me to go home and get on with life.

By mid-November I could barely eat and my stomach became increasingly bloated. I was admitted to the hospital—reluctantly the day before Thanksgiving. It looked like normal life might be ending for me. In the crisis, my family kicked in again and made yet another holiday memory: We all had Thanksgiving dinner together the weekend before the real holiday would take place. After I was admitted, Mom, Dad, and Greg shared a quiet and not-quite-home-cooked meal in the Florida Hospital cafeteria on the traditional "Family Day of Thanks." Florida Hospital is surrounded by some very beautiful topography. Greg and Mom spent part of the day walking through the trees along the lake, hoping to blow off some stress we all felt as the doctors searched in vain for a solution.

The doctors let me go home the first week of December (2004). I had been through two separate procedures: a cholecystectomy (gallbladder removal) and the insertion of a jejunostomy tube (or "J" tube). From this point forward most of my daily nutrition would be delivered through that tube in my gut. After a relatively brief stint at home, I was back in the hospital and not released again until the day before Christmas Eve. Christmas Day my family joined hands and offered up prayers of gratefulness not only for the birth of Christ, but that I had been able to come home. With so many problems and so few answers, we were reaching a point where not one of us was sure if I would come home from the hospital the next time.

In March, 2005, I started noticing some changes in my blood sugar levels. Eighty is ideal, and I was starting to see higher numbers. I told no one and shrugged it off on the cookies. Denial again. The morning I hit 126, however, I freaked out. Something *was* wrong with the pancreas. My blood sugar levels soon crept into the 200s, then 300s, and finally to almost 500. We discussed it at length with the doctors, but they simply shook their heads. The pancreas had failed. Nothing could be done to save it.

I was a full-fledged type 1 diabetic again. *Oh dear God, what now?*

At first I was shocked and confused. It just didn't compute in my head. What could possibly be the purpose behind getting such a short glimpse of normal life? I had temporarily tasted a fairly regular existence. I had no worries about blood sugars, no shots, no fear of seizures, or damaging my kidney any further. I just couldn't comprehend why this still new gift would be taken away.

> There was nothing to be done except cry again, fill syringes with insulin, and stick them in my body again, and again, and again.

When I was finally able to accept the facts, anger flooded in. Through clenched teeth I began a sort of bargaining process with God. I thought that maybe my prayers hadn't been specific enough. I had asked for a normal life, but I hadn't asked Him for a normal life for *the rest* of my life. Maybe He misunderstood; maybe if I asked again.

My sister Karen wrestled deeply with the "why" questions too. All she had ever known was a diabetic sister. And then, for almost two years, all of us had a season of relative normalcy (and lots of Krispy Kreme donuts). She confesses, "I loved that time for Linda. I had prayed for the miracle of the non-diabetic life for my sister for so long. For a while we had it. We were living in the moment, the moment where we could proclaim, 'Yes! It's true! Miracles happen! Amen to the answered prayer!' and then it evaporated. For the life of me, I can't figure out what benefit has come from losing that pancreas."

Even today, the loss pushes me to the edge of my faith. I simply don't understand the purpose behind losing that pancreas either; I cannot find the good in it at all. I hope and I pray that I will be receptive enough to listen and understand when God tells me why. Perhaps, someday, I will understand the purpose behind that brief season of a more normal life. But for now, I just don't get it.

It took a long time for my tears to dry. When they did, I could clearly see reality: I was walking in the valley of the shadow of death.

I looked into the possibility of a second pancreas transplant but the risks and complications were just too high. There was nothing to be done except cry again, fill syringes with insulin, and stick them in my body again, and again, and again.

Oh, it was so very hard to return to all of the concerns and logistics and fears of a diabetic life. Physical life changes were significant, to say the least. The hardest transition, though, had to take place in my soul: I had to accept that the pink fog is real after all and it was getting closer. For the first time my health had taken an irreversible step in the wrong direction and there was nothing I could do about it. I was stepping backwards instead of going forward. I didn't have any other options. I had had brushes with death before, but now I had to face the truth that death was not a matter of *if*, it was only a matter of *when*.

That year I developed a number of ulcers on my heel and some of my toes. They bled constantly. They still do. Greg says it's like being married to Gretel—I leave a trail of blood spots behind me. It is a symptom of poor circulation. Prolonged pressure on my feet causes the skin to crack open, exposing me to infection and gangrene (and that spells a-m-p-u-t-a-t-i-o-n for a diabetic). On top of that was the continued degradation of the nerves to my peripheral and autonomic system. The numbness I have from the upper hips all the way down meant I was prone to falling. And should I injure myself, I can't feel it and I'm likely to cause more damage. Walking also meant consistent sharp stabbing and burning pain when the nerves were stimulated. Severe pain in my right hip after my kidney transplant was the new organ resting partially just inside the upper pocket of the pelvic/hip region. In short, the more I walked, the worse the pain and numbness became and the more I exposed myself to further injury. Another reality check. Another difficult decision. It wasn't a choice, really. I had no other option. I began to navigate the world from the confines of a wheelchair.

The failure of the pancreas and the reality of the wheelchair were all pointing in the wrong direction. Physically I slumped into fatigue. Emotionally I slid from discouragement into depression. In the darkness of my room, under the cover of sleep, I hid from the inevitable end. It took a long time for my tears to dry. When they did, I could clearly see reality: I was walking in the valley of the shadow of death.

The valley became deeper and darker on February 26, 2006. I was having an "off day." Lying in bed I felt dizzy and had a hard time seeing—neither of these was uncommon, but something else was happening, something I'd never experienced before. It seemed like I was looking into a bright halogen light and all I could hear was a rushing sound in my ears—like water surging through my head—yet I could hear no sound in the room. Breathing was very, very difficult, intensely difficult, as if a heavy, heavy blanket had been laid upon my body. I was struggling so hard that in my mind I began to wrestle with the possibility that breathing was no longer worth the effort. It would be so easy to just surrender, to give up the fight. At the same time, however, vivid thoughts of loved ones swirled in my mind. *If you give up, you'll never get to see, feel, or touch Greg again. Everything you share with your parents will come to an end, and Karen would become an only child. You will miss out on so much.*

I started fighting for consciousness and breath. I reached for the phone that Greg always leaves near my hand when he leaves the house. Miraculously, Greg happened to look down and see the light of his cell phone flashing while he was on an ellipse machine at the gym. He could barely hear me; I had so little air to spare for words. He rushed from the gym and jumped in his car, screaming at me through the phone as he drove. Dashing into the house he found me on the bed soaked in sweat, drained of color, fading in and out of consciousness.

A call to 911, frantic words with the emergency dispatcher, the EMTs, familiar faces, who were used to emergencies at our home. They believed that I was going through some sort of an overdose or medication imbalance and transported me by ambulance to the hospital.

I don't remember much after that. Fading in and out of consciousness, the world seemed hazy around the edges. Fuzzy images of people moved back and forth, their voices echoing unclearly. I began to hear a horrible growling sound, like a dog, very base, but it wasn't an animal; it was me trying to let them know I couldn't breathe—I couldn't breathe.

In the ER the doctors and the emergency team were talking about my medications when the nurses became frantic: *blood pressure dropping, respirations dissipating, and no pulse.* I was crashing. The next thing Greg knew there were six people at my bed working frantically; others yelled instructions to others who ran for equipment and meds. Brian O'Connell, a male nurse, was doing full chest compressions with his 6'2", 225-pound body.

> Greg clenched his fists and shouted, "She cannot die! She cannot die!"

Greg collapsed in front of the nurses' station sobbing. Linda Kasen (an angel who only disguises herself as a nurse) and others scooped him off the floor and moved him to a room where they tried to calm him down. "Everything is going to be okay," they told him. "God's grace is going to be with you. It's going to be with Linda. It's going to be with your family." Greg clenched his fists and shouted, "She cannot die! She cannot die!"

But Greg was wrong. I could die. And I did.

My heart stopped for a full three minutes. The doctors did everything they could. Linda Kasen saw that I was blue from head to toe. She had seen this plenty of times in her career. Knowing that hearing is the last sense to fail during any functional breakdown, she got in my face and yelled at me to hold on. "Don't give up! Don't you give up!" And louder still through her tears, "Don't you *dare* give up!"

I woke up in the Cardiac ICU around two o'clock the next morning. I could hear talking and a few familiar voices—Greg, my mom, my dad—but I couldn't quite get my brain around what had happened. They told me the story, but it just didn't soak in to my mind. The words "cardiac arrest" just didn't compute. The thought that my heart had stopped was so scary I just kind of hung my brain in mental limbo—not really blocking it out, but not accepting it as being fact, either.

Emotions swirled through my soul. Thankfulness, anger, pain, relief, but above them all, a new terrifying fear of being alone. Part of me wanted to leave this hospital so I could be by myself. I wanted to be home in my closet where I felt safe, where no one could bother me and where I could say whatever I wanted to for as long as I needed. Another part of me knew that if I left the hospital and the care of all of those around me, I would certainly die.

Dying alone. The thought descended with terror. Another cardiac arrest could happen. What if I were alone?! What if no one was there to call 911? What if I never get to say goodbye? What if the next time my family sees me, I'm dead? *I can't be alone. I can't be alone.*

Greg has always felt responsible to protect me, and he wrestled with this from the other side. "The thought of leaving her alone for any period of time was incomprehensible; someone had to be with her constantly. Bonnie and Karl and I tried to work out a schedule to make that work, but if Linda was to have any quality of life, if she was to have any long-term sanity, she had to have some time to herself, just like we did."

I prayed and prayed and prayed for a solution. I asked God for peace. I wanted something calming to wash over me and let me know that it was okay to be alone. If I had just thought about it long enough, I would have realized that God had already given me the answer. He had already put it out there; I just couldn't see the big picture yet.

A month later Greg and I were still having a hard time believing that I had been through a full cardiac arrest. It was hard to imagine that anything like that would happen again. But on March 25, while we were hanging out in our living room, I started to feel unusually tired. Greg made fun of me as I nodded off with my mouth hanging open.

Then he suddenly jumped to attention. He recalls, "She started making these horrible gasping noises and her eyes rolled back in her head. I thought, *Oh no, this is not happening again; there is no way this is happening again.* I ran over to her and shook her and yelled, 'Linda! What's wrong!' She said, 'I'm okay, I'm just having a moment.'" This was one of the lame things I would say to nicely let Greg know I wanted to be left alone. I always thought that phrase would do it, but he'd heard it too many times before to fall for it now, especially now!

"She started to lose consciousness," he recalls. "I shook her; I slapped her right across the face. All of a sudden—and I've never seen anything like this in my life—her eyes went off in all directions. I call it the 'Marty Feldman' eyes . . . totally goofy, but also blank and empty—no light in them at all. Linda turned ghost white. And then she stopped breathing."

A call to 911, frantic words with the emergency dispatcher, and Greg wrestled with my limp body, trying to position it in a way that would help me breathe. Finally a low guttural moan escaped my lips. The EMTs arrived, throwing chairs and pushing tables out of the way. They found a pulse and quickly tried to assess my situation, but these were not the familiar faces we knew, and "my situation" is not very simple. Greg gave them a copy of my medical history and a list of the medicines I was taking. (We keep these papers ready for an emergency.) Overwhelmed by the length of the list, they started questioning me about some of the medications, assuming that maybe I was going through some sort of an overdose. But I wasn't. It was my heart, again. In the ambulance I was placed in physical restraints as I struggled to breathe and battled for consciousness. I was fighting and growling again, but I knew I was defenseless from every angle. In the ER they cut off my négligée (Greg's favorite and mine too), along with my last sense of dignity and decency. I was completely exposed to all who walked by. I couldn't feel much, but everything I did feel felt compromised, violated, vulnerable.

> It was well with my soul, but my body was still in bad shape.

They stabilized me and moved me to the CICU where more tests were started. A steady flow of doctors moved in and out of my room as I settled in for a nine-day recovery. I was discharged with two IV antibiotics and one oral one, but it was clear that they were not working. As Gomer Pyle used to say; "Surprise, surprise, surprise!" Readmitted again to Florida Hospital Orlando, the doctors worked on some new issues as well as some leftover ones. Several days later Greg was trying to catch up at work. He was suddenly overcome with a powerful sense of dread. Something was wrong, but he didn't know what it was. He tried to call my hospital room in the Progressive Care Unit (PCU). The phone rang and rang; no one picked it up. The nurses' station offered him little information. All they knew at the moment was that something had happened and that a doctor and several nurses were in my room. Greg raced from his office and drove as fast as he reasonably could. Along the way he called his parents to let them know that something was very, very wrong with me. My mom finally reached him by cell phone as he pulled into the hospital parking garage. She told him what the doctor's had said, confirming what he already knew in his heart: "Linda is really scary right now; things are really scary," she said.

My mom had been staying with me that day and I was hurting pretty bad. In the process of giving me CPR during the first cardiac arrest, Brian O'Connell had broken three of my ribs. I never imagined that I would be grateful to the man who beat me up so badly, but I really was. He was another person who had saved my life. While I lay in bed, the rib pain was overshadowed by now familiar sensations. *Oh my God, it's happening again.* My mom yelled for help as I struggled for breath. One of the nurses called Dr. Crockett, who had asked me over the phone to describe the symptoms I was experiencing. "Help me; help me," was all I could whisper. He dropped what he was doing and started running from that part of the hospital campus across the street.

They rushed my bed towards the ICU, and we "just happened" to run into my cardiologist, Dr. Joel D. Greenberg. He was the first of a long stream of people that God brought to us precisely when we needed them the most. Miraculously, my dad drove through the middle of town during rush hour and was never slowed by traffic; he didn't have to stop for a single red light. "It was like the Red Sea parting for Moses," he said. Friends showed up and began praying with Greg and my mom. Even Dr. Des Cummings Jr., Executive VP of Florida Hospital and the President of the FH Foundation, rushed to our side.

When Dr. Crockett arrived, he caught up to the lot of us racing down the corridors. Running beside my bed, he leaned over, placed his cheek against my cheek and began whispering reassurances. "It's going to be okay. It's going to be okay . . . ."

"Help me; help me. I can't breathe," was all I could whisper. In the ICU, Dr. Greenberg was cheek to cheek with me on the other side, lovingly and caringly stroking my forehead and holding my hand. I could feel the strength in his grip; he wasn't going to let go for anything, but he was also screaming at the nurses, "Get me another amp of atropine!" Then he whispered in my ear, "I'm not going to let anything happen to you." In the midst of the commotion, I found myself in the closet of my soul one more time. *Please dear God—let them keep their promises. Please. I am giving this to You my precious Lord and Savior. I know now more than ever You will not let me go nor will You let me down.*

In that moment, with both of these dear men so close to me, I began to feel a peace beyond the circumstances. I felt comfortable, comfortable for the first time in a long, long time. I was in the best possible hands and felt I could release and begin letting things happen to me. I had never felt that before; I had always felt the need to fight, but this time the fight belonged to someone else. Everyone I needed was there—Greg, my parents, a very dear and special friend, and the best doctors. I was relieved I just didn't need to be in control anymore. I *wasn't* in control, and for the first time ever, that didn't scare me at all. It was well with my soul, but my body was still in bad shape.

As I was prepped and wheeled into the OR, my family and friends were told to say a quick "Good-bye." Dr. Des Cummings Jr., and Dr. Crockett watched the entire procedure from the observation window of the OR. They were the only two human beings looking down and watching over me, but they were not alone, either. "Where two or more are gathered, I will also be there," Jesus promised.

Dr. Greenberg was certain that he was merely minutes from some level of serious open chest/heart surgery. He began a cardiac catheterization. When Des came down to see my family in the waiting room, it was the first time they had ever seen him truly scared. The family and friends who arrived formed a circle of prayer along with several of the hospital staff.

When Dr. Greenberg came out, he told them that I was stable, but he was not even cautiously optimistic. He diagnosed me with cardiomyopathy. The muscles of my heart had stiffened and could not respond to even minute changes in heart rhythm and balance. This is not a problem that can be fixed by surgery. Treatment would take place over time through more medicine. A permanent pacemaker might be required. I was just forty years old and had essentially no immune system—not a stellar combination along with all of my other challenges.

It was a sober moment. I felt I was deep in the valley, having narrowly escaped the pink fog one more time. But it wasn't all darkness. When everything settled down, Dr. Greenberg gave me

> I know what is waiting for me on the other side, Paradise. I'm just not ready yet.

some of the most sensible and realistic advice that I've ever received in my life. He said, "Linda, This can happen again. Next time, you might go too far for us to bring you back. It could happen ten days from now. It could happen ten years from now. It could even happen more than ten years from now. We will give these meds time to do the job they are meant to do. Your job is to enjoy life as much as you possibly can. Go to the movies. Have a good time. Go out to dinner. Have a big steak and a double martini."

A big steak and a double martini . . . .

I have to admit, it's a little unnerving when the best advice that one of the best cardiologists in the world can give you is to go load up on red meat and alcohol. But I understand exactly what he meant. I believe he thought a double martini might just be able to fix at least something that ailed me, because I had a choice at this point: *Would I only wait to die? Or would I choose to live?*

For months the shadow of death had hung over me like the fog of my nightmare. I wondered if each breath might not be my last. I feared that every heartbeat might be followed by another flat line. In the midst of the emergencies, I wasn't able to say anything; I didn't know what was going on; I was totally out of control of the situation. At that moment I didn't have the capacity to choose whether or not I was going to live or die, and that scared me terribly.

My heart and mind and soul so desperately want to be here with my family and the other people that I love and care for, but I am not afraid to die. I know what is waiting for me on the other side, Paradise. I'm just not ready yet. The amazing people in my blessed life have made my life here on this side just too much fun to want to leave the party . . . yet. I believe that I am still here to help and to serve people—but my will to live (strong as it might be) has limitations. When the time comes to face death again, I might not be the one that gets to make a choice. Instead of getting to choose between staying and letting go, I might actually forcibly die.

I feared being alone after the first cardiac arrest. God made it clear after the second and third episodes that *if He chooses to do so,* He can surround me with all the help my body needs to survive. Ultimately, however, it doesn't matter if I'm surrounded by twenty doctors or if I'm completely alone. When physical death draws near for the last time, medical decisions may rest in the hands of the nurses and doctors, but, ultimately, my destiny is in God's hands alone, a God who will never leave me alone. When it's my time to go, it's my time to go. My "job" is to live wisely within my illnesses, but I am certainly not to live fearfully. I am to live fully.

Many years ago, in 1984, it was the night before very scary surgery and complete darkness filled my hospital room and my entire life. I had lost my sight completely on February 16, 1984. Both of my retinas had been damaged and blood from many small and some larger vessels had filled the cavity in the rear of my eyes. The only light I could sense came when very bright light was aimed directly into the eye. It looked deep, an intense magenta pink.

Dr. Chambers performed another vitrectomy. Making numerous incisions in my eye, he drained the blood-infused fluid and replaced it with a new artificial fluid. The future of my sight hung in the balance.

It was a "closet moment." If I had had the opportunity, I would have loved to have felt the security within the boundaries of those four walls. In the hospital room, the best I could do was imagine being completely alone with God. I did, and began to take my concerns and my fears to Him. Mid-prayer I fell asleep, my conscious requests to God mixing in a dream. In the dream I became very aware of my fear and nervousness. As I did, I began to see the world around me engulfed in a sparkling white—like the snow of a perfect Christmas morning. No color, no sound, just whiteness. At first I thought this meant I was going blind; the surgery would not be a success. I started to panic. But this whiteness was different. It was a glowing, perfect light. I started to feel something different: I was warmed by this light, and the more I took it in, the more comfort I felt. Fear evaporated and calm descended; this was the presence of God, coming to me, letting me know that I would be okay. No matter what happened, I was going to be okay, because I was not alone.

When physical death draws near for the last time, medical decisions may rest in the hands of the nurses and doctors, but, ultimately, my destiny is in God's hands alone, a God who will never leave me alone.

Whether this dream was just in my mind or whether it was some sort of real reflection of spiritual and physical realities, I will probably never know. Regardless, the dream gave me a picture of a truth—a truth that is not hard to understand, even though it is sometimes very difficult to believe. But believe it we must, for when we feel alone, when the pink fog pursues us relentlessly, we must stand on what is real:

Though I walk through the valley of the shadow of death, I fear no evil; for Thou art with me. (Psalm 23:4)

Even though He slay me,
yet I will trust Him.

~ Job 13:15

Perhaps God gives us difficulties in order to give us the opportunity to know who we really are and who we really can be. We live in a world that is sometimes constipated by its own superficiality. But life's difficulties are even a privilege, in that they allow us or force us to break through the superficiality to the deeper life within.

Me in the Mirror

10

I WAS STANDING IN FRONT OF THE MIRROR the other day, taking inventory of the image reflected back. It was pretty sobering. From head to toe the body I saw told story after story, like a veteran's journal chronicling war battles. It was a strange sensation, really, to look at that body in the mirror. I felt detached and yet inseparable from what's left of the flesh and bones before me. Someday I'll be separated from that body. The walk through the valley of the shadow of death taught me that. *When that happens, what will be left? Who am I? When I look in the mirror, who is it that is looking back?*

> *This is the suffering of a healthy person, as undramatic as it is inevitable, as commonplace as it is uncomforted. It is the pain with a thousand private faces, the pain that comes from just being human. No man is inoculated against the ache of his struggle to become himself as a*

human being and a child of God.[28]

Eugene Kennedy

God uses hardship and pain—like carving tools in the hands of a master carpenter. He strips away, shaving by shaving, who I am not. He shapes me into the authentically human and fully aware child of God I'm supposed to be.

Let's face it, our entire society measures us by what we *look like*, what we *possess* and what we *do*. When I'm honest, I see that each of these can become a superficial façade—masks that have nothing to do with who I truly am. An accident, an injury, or the continual nagging of a chronic degenerative disease strips away at that superficial lie to reveal who it really is that looks back from the mirror.

Joni Eareckson Tada learned this the hard way. Months after her broken neck, she was still strapped down on a revolving gurney when two high school classmates came to visit her. When they saw her face, one of them ran from the room and puked while the other sobbed loudly. Joni insisted someone bring her a mirror:

> *The figure in the mirror seemed scarcely human. As I stared at my own reflection, I saw two eyes, darkened and sunk into the sockets, bloodshot and glassy . . . . I appeared to be little more than a skeleton covered by yellow, jaundiced skin. My shaved head only accented my grotesque skeletal appearance. As I talked, I saw my teeth, black from the effects of the medication. I too felt like vomiting.*[29]

Joni's disfigurement was the result of a traumatic accident. Though she remains paralyzed, her appearance got better. In my opinion, she has aged beautifully. My situation is a little bit different. It's been a slow slide downhill. When it comes to appearances—what I look like—the cut of God's chisel on my body has been very real as decades and disease have done their work.

The photos reproduced in the middle of this book show this process a lot better than I could describe it in words. But here's the way I experienced it. The slide started pretty simply. At first I just didn't like the way my old clothes hung on me, but then again, I didn't like the way *I* hung on me. Now I look like a zipper project from some middle school home economics assignment gone insane. So far, I have accumulated nearly five feet of scars. I have two extra organs on one side of my torso and tubes sticking in and out of me on the other. My bloated stomach makes me look pregnant, and under my slinky negligees I wear some really sexy Depends underwear. (Let's just say that Victoria's Secret doesn't call for photo-ops very often.) Today if I ask, "Mirror, mirror on the wall, who is the fairest of them all?" the mirror cracks up laughing.

I know in my head that beauty is more than skin deep, but it's really tough to convince my ego of that. How I see myself, inside and out, affects every interaction I have out there in the world, and it deeply affects how I relate to Greg. Time has proven that he loves me with supernatural agape love, but I wasn't secure in that at first. Even back when my body had all its curves in the right places, I was terrified about seizures—but not for medical reasons, it was much more emotional. *What will Greg think of me if he sees me thrashing around out of control?* I didn't want him to see my body contorting in all those horrible ways, making all those really awful sounds. *Will he think less of me as a woman? Will I be less attractive to him sexually? Will the passion still be there?* I was concerned that something I couldn't control would somehow change the way that he saw me. Would he see me differently after watching me disappear into a grand mal seizure? Just the possibility that he might reject me made me mad. *If this makes me unattractive then, that's not fair. I can't help it so why would he feel that way?!*

It's really that mirror's fault. The "me in the mirror" is a real shock and a real disappointment. When I look at myself in the mirror, I think, *Wow, that's not the way I really want to look for Greg.* Long gone are the days when a slender, sleek, elegant, beautiful, sexy woman greeted him at the door. It's just not candlelight and curves like we dreamed it would be. I don't like the way I look and don't look the way I want to for Greg, a very tough mixture of wanting it for him and wanting it for myself.

The feelings about my body and feelings about how my husband feels about my body are unavoidable issues in the wake of all I have been through. These are normal fears for anyone; it just seems turned up full steam because of disease and injury. I guess it's similar to the expected aging process; it just feels like the process has been stuck on fast forward way too long.

To make matters worse, the reflection in the mirror is more distorted because I feel so lousy all the time. The feedback my brain gets from my body screams "Houston, we have a problem. Eject!" The mirror tells me I look like Frankenstein— though I don't have a scar all the way around my neck . . . yet. (But hmmm, maybe that's not a bad idea. If I could keep my head and get a whole-body transplant . . . . I'll have to call my doctor on that one.)

Who am I? If my true identity depends on how I feel and how I look, I'm in deep trouble.

The manure pile of self-image gets even deeper when I consider what I have—that is, my possessions. Yes, I know, "There aren't any U-hauls behind a hearse." I also know, "He who dies with the most toys . . . still dies." Money and possessions aren't everything, but they are something. Insurance hassles, lost income, and this big black hole of medical expenses have made it very, very tough to get through the end of the month. I try to completely trust God all the time in everything, but honestly, none of us do that very well. No human is capable of complete trust in anyone or anything, no matter what they say. We are always clinging to the desire to have at least a little bit of control—and in our culture, control equals money.

Our special talents also help define us for the world. One of my greatest senses of loss came when I lost my voice. I can still talk, of course, but I used to be able to sing. *Really* sing. When my voice gave way, so did something in my heart. The loss was almost incalculable, a true closet moment. *God, this makes no sense at all. Why in the world would you strip me of something that I used to praise you?* I still don't get that one, but I'm coming to believe that it has something to do with discovering who I truly am. It's one more thing stripped away, showing me that whoever I am, I'm not the girl with the lovely voice anymore. The voice that once could bring tears to most of my audience, even some men, now brings forth tears from a different audience: me. I still miss the ability to be special. I yearn for the chance to sing for others and to use that beautiful God-given gift to sing of His glory, grace, and mercy.

And money relates to what we *do*. Does what I do define who I am? No, that doesn't help at all. My abilities to perform in the world have been pretty much a one-way, downhill street. When Greg and I got married, I had an okay job that helped pay the rent. Greg had joined the insurance company just seven weeks after I got my position. My dad worked there his entire career. Granddaddy, my dad's dad, worked there his entire career. When I started in February 1994, Dad gave me a corporate plate that Granddaddy had given him—a passing of the professional torch. I attacked my work with the expectation of living up to the family legacy and even surpassing it. Then my ship came in. In a new position at a prestigious insurance company, my career took off like crazy. In January of 2000 we were seriously thinking about selling our new house and moving to Chicago so I could climb the corporate ladder even faster. I was a picture of perfect health and the sky was the limit. Then February 16, 2000, rolled around. The impact of that major stroke shook my health like an earthquake hitting a house of cards. The company just wouldn't put up with my absences due to medical illness. When I was let go, I was overcome with a tremendous sense of failure. I felt like I had let everyone down.

> *What will Greg think of me if he sees me thrashing around out of control? I didn't want him to see my body contorting in all those horrible ways, making all those really awful sounds.*

Who was the woman in the mirror the next morning? All I knew was that she wasn't a big-wig corporate insurance exec.

The wheelchair hasn't helped either. It creates an obscure barrier between me and the rest of humanity. Some people seem to deal with it okay, but the chair makes others feel uneasy and self-conscious, insulating me and cutting me off from a regular flow of relationships. People treat me like I'm invisible or mentally handicapped. Sometimes people ignore me or ask questions about me to the person accompanying me, as if I have no brain in my head. Maybe they think I am unable to speak for myself. Do they think that if my legs don't work my brain doesn't either? I guess there are many reasons for being treated like this, but I get pretty tired of being defined by that chair. How much better would be if we all could reach across the barrier of illness and disease and touch each other as real people!

What I can and can't do clearly affects my relationship with Greg, too. Physical challenges are a definite challenge to physical intimacy. The barriers come in many forms. The smells, the oxygen tank, the IV pump, even our bed is broken into two sections that move independently of each other, making it nearly impossible to snuggle. I don't care what anyone says; it's a struggle when physical intimacy is disrupted. When someone says that's the least important part of marriage, they either don't know or don't care. We've been married sixteen years now and it's still pretty important to me. Ask me on our 50th anniversary and I'll tell you if it's still in the top three, but right now it's still pretty close to the top!

I miss the unhindered, spontaneous expressions of our love for each other. That is the main way I can share something with my husband that nobody else gets. It's been taken away on the outside. The me that I want him to have is still there on the inside, but it's been scarred, too. The cuts have been so deep on the outside that my insides have all sorts of scars, too. How I feel about myself changes the way I relate to him. Giving and receiving on this level is really important, but now the body that I want to give him no longer exists.

These struggles test the boundaries of human love. God has given me such an incredibly understanding and selfless spouse. I know that many aren't nearly so lucky. He puts up with all my meds and moods and diapers and barf-buckets without a complaint—and he still kisses me first thing when he gets home in the evening. What he tolerates is unbelievable.

Daily, God strips away at Greg, as well. I wish it wasn't so; and I wish it wasn't because of me. I believe that there are certain earthly rewards for people like him—an inner God-given fulfillment. But I also believe that Greg will receive the full kick-back for what he chooses to do in eternity.

But what does all this do to Greg's identity? Who does he see when he looks in the mirror? Sometimes the relationship gets a little blurry:

> It's been really tough to focus on Linda as my wife rather than seeing her as my patient. It's hard to separate that sometimes. It's easy to become mechanical and clinical toward the illness. Those feelings get transferred to the person. I have to fight to keep that from happening, and I've got to do it all the time, or that can become the direction that the marriage takes . . . . I refuse to be defined by the caretaker roll. Sure, this disease shapes us into what we are; but we are not this disease. I'm a husband first . . . always—except when she's convulsing. Then I transform into an amazingly dashing paramedic.

We've found that there is no substitute for personal time together. Greg has never lost the art of dating. That has kept us thriving and not just surviving. Dinner, a movie, a walk around the block on a beautiful day—not only are they good for our relationship, but they are defiant acts of rebellion against the disease. They prove that as long as we have breath we will prevail, celebrate, and live it up. We've found our own versions of the steak and martini that Dr. Greenberg ordered, and it works when we choose to seize the moment and capture the day.

Creativity and commitment in the context of open communication keep a vital stream of intimate affirmation flowing, even when physical barriers seem insurmountable. It takes work, but this is marriage—a continual adjustment of two lives becoming one, an ongoing mix-up that blends our lives into one. The first time we tried to share our denominational backgrounds it almost killed my dad. Greg is Episcopalian; my parents are hardcore Presbyterian. Back in the day, when Greg was still trying to win over my dad, they were walking down the aisle at our church when Greg suddenly stopped and genuflected (a quick kneel towards the altar as a sign of reverence). Dad never expected that and he tripped right over Greg . . . right there in the middle of church, right in front of God and everyone.

Greg and my dad worked out their differences, and Greg and I agree that we will always talk about our struggles—even if it is three o'clock in the morning and he needs to get up for work the next day. If you truly love a person, there's always a way to find both physical and emotional attraction. (Or maybe it's the other way around: Maybe true love comes from a willingness to always find a way.) We keep the option of counseling open, too. Although our journey is uniquely ours, we know we aren't the first to go through it. This is the rhythm of the generations of humanity. We are simply learning to dance to it in our own special way.

Yes, we are shaped by what we have been through, but it does not define us. We have a drama, but we're not letting it take over our lives or overshadow our family. It's not easy. Nothing worthwhile comes easily. But we don't let anyone feel sorry for us as if we're suffering in some way. We know we are a family; things happen for a reason; we will figure it out and we will get through it all together. Illness forces us to dig deep beneath the physical surface to find that person that we truly love, to discover who we really are, and it has allowed us to discover the kind of intimacy that we dreamed of sharing and receiving in the first place.

One day I was really struggling with my lingering sex-appeal, our financial struggles, and the things I just couldn't do anymore. I was ready to give up and call it quits. My body has changed in just about every way and place possible. I was positive that I wasn't sexy to anyone, even my own husband. But then Greg scooped me up in his arms, wiped away my tears and said, "Dead isn't sexy," and gave me a big old smooch. I was positive that I couldn't love him any more than I did at that moment.

Okay, back to the question: Who is that in the mirror? If my identity is not based on my appearance, my possessions or my abilities, then who am I?

In relation to this, my prayers regularly sounded like a combination of *begging* and *anger*. They were often confused and exhausting. I did a lot of searching through my Bible to make sure that those kinds of prayers were okay. I was relieved to find out that Job, David, and Moses all felt the freedom to vent their true emotions to God. Even Jesus raised His eyes to heaven in His deepest hour of need and cried, "Father, why have you abandoned me?!" So I entered the closet yet again and found my voice in prayers that were angry, thankful, sad, and demanding, all at the same time.

What it all comes down to is this:

Either God exists or He doesn't. If there is an all-powerful, all-present, all-loving personal being, then He alone can tell me who I am. When all hell seems to cut loose and I'm in the process of losing it all, only He has the perspective that can bring peace and purpose into the mix and show me who I really am. Isaiah 40:6-8 lays it out like this:

> Shout that people are like the grass that dies away. Their beauty fades as quickly as the beauty of flowers in a field. The grass withers and the flowers fade beneath the breath of the Lord. And so it is with people. The grass withers and the flowers fade, but the word of our God stands forever (NLT).

That's pretty clear. My outward beauty fades; my physical life withers. God's Word, however, stands forever. So forget the mirror, the Bible is where I must look to find a true reflection of who I am. And what does His everlasting Word say about me?

- ✧ I am loved. (Romans 8:38-39)

- ✧ God looks at the heart, not my outward appearance. (2 Samuel 16:11)

- ✧ Earthly possessions don't last; they don't matter at all. (Matthew 6:19-20)

- ✧ I am accepted regardless of my performance. (Ephesians 2:8-9)

- ✧ I have hope. (Psalm 27:13)

- ✧ I am God's child. (1 John 3:1-2)

- ✧ While my earthly existence will become increasingly

difficult and painful, beyond the grave I will experience the power and perfection of a body that will never, never be sick again. (1 Corinthians 15:35-44) *I like this one!*

✧ The day is coming when I will have no more pain, tears, or regrets. None. (Revelation 21:4) I really like the *no more pain* part in this one, too!

I am really living in a shadow. It is a real shadow and I will never minimize how dark it is. But where there is darkness there is a light—I just need to be willing to see it. Through my disease I have been given a preview of the complete physical loss that every member of humanity will experience, most of them after it's too late to change the focus of their lives. I have been given the opportunity to refuse the façade and become real, *today*.

As Joni Eareckson Tada stabilized from her paralyzing accident, she also began to recover from the mental and emotional trauma that tormented her soul. One day, a close friend even dared suggest that her paralysis might be a blessing. Joni resisted the idea, but her friend was gently persistent, and appealed to her sense as an artist to make his point. "Joni, your body, in the chair—is only the frame for God's portrait of you. Y'know, people don't go to an art gallery to admire frames. Their focus is on the quality and character of the painting," he said. Joni's response was:

This made sense. I could relax and not worry so much about my appearance. God was "painting" me in just the perfect way so I could enhance the character of Christ within. This gave a whole new perspective to the chair. Once it had been a terrible burden, a trial for me. Then, as I saw God working in my life, it became only a tool. Now, I could see it as a blessing. For the first time in my paralyzed life, it was indeed possible for that wheelchair to be an instrument of joy in my life.[30]

A wheelchair as an instrument of joy? That hardly seems possible to me. Or does it? God is using my diabetes as an instrument to strip away who I am not. Can He use it to reveal who I am in Him? If so, then I can draw an even more radical conclusion: *My disease can be, in part, viewed as a gift . . . something to be thankful for.* Joni came to the same conclusion:

In the days that followed, I thanked him for "me"—whatever I was in terms of mind, spirit, personality—and even my body. I thank him for the way I looked and for what I could do and could not do. As I did, the doctrine of his sovereignty helped everything fall into place, like a jigsaw puzzle. Not only was there purpose to my life at this point, but there was an iceberg of potential as well—10% above the surface, 90% below. It was an exciting thought—an entire new era of my life and personality not even developed yet.[30]

One time I asked Greg when was the last time that he had thanked God for something good that was coming out of all the struggles we faced. He confessed that he was so angry about some of the things that were happening that he couldn't remember the last time he had given thanks. I asked them to do me a favor—to do himself a favor—and take the time to make some thanks. He did; we did, and as a result we began to discover not only who we truly are as individuals but who we are as a married couple becoming one in a real, rather than superficial, way.

In light of who God claims to be, He commands me to give thanks, even in the depths of darkness (1 Thessalonians 5:18), even for the things I can't do, for the things I have lost, and for my fading beauty. It's a huge step of faith, but freedom and joy greet me on the other side every time I choose to move in that direction. God is using my disease to remove the superficial and reveal who I really am. By faith and by hope I can find blessings and give thanks in spite of who I see in the mirror— if I choose to do so. That's a step of faith unlike any other. Oftentimes it means opening my mouth to give thanks before I know what it is I can be thankful for. But item by item my list of blessings grows, a list of powerfully real things, things that reach deep into the soul of our humanity and touch us where we long to be touched. It's a miracle, actually. Every time I choose to look beyond the surface and embrace the deeper things, faith triumphs over feelings as biblical truth conquers the lie of the mirror.

Indeed, medical problems have made me the person that I am, and I'm proud of the person than I am. Those medical problems have taught me things that I otherwise might never have learned or come to appreciate. They shape me and mold me into something better. And so I have to be thankful for the pain along with the laugher, the decay along with the hope, because that is who I am. When I look in that mirror I really wouldn't change a thing.

Well, except maybe for my bloated stomach. I hate my bloated stomach.

That is why we never give up. Though our bodies are dying, our inner person is being renewed every day. For our present troubles are quite small and won't last very long. Yet they produce for us an immeasurably great glory that will last forever! So we don't look at the troubles we can see right now; rather we look forward to what we have not yet seen. For the troubles we see will soon be over, but the joys to come will last forever.

2 Corinthians 4:16-18 (NLT)

But the question in the midst of all this is how can we, knowing that life is so incredibly delicious and short-lived, still continue to live bland, insipid lives? . . . how can we keep on indefinitely preparing to live, knowing that each day comes but once in human history?

~ Tim Hansel

If Today
is all
I Have

11

*T*HE WORDS SOUNDED DISTANT AND FAMILIAR—too familiar. "Please know that there has been no mistake." The words of a doctor in a white coat echoing across the decades, resonating as they did the day my family came to the end of the white picket fence.

"Please know that there has been no mistake."

Greg and I sat listening, understanding what was said—but unable to comprehend. They were simple words that didn't quite compute; answers that weren't unexpected, just shocking. *After all these years, I should be an expert at this—at getting bad news.*

But it was a different kind of news that day, different from every meeting with every doctor since that day the six-year-old girl's parents were told that the needle would be her way of life. Greg and I listened as the doctor used phrases like, *I'm sorry. I can't give you cardiac clearance. I'm sorry. I don't know where we go from here. I'm sorry. There is nothing left for us to do.*

I don't know where we go from here. I'm sorry. There is nothing left for us to do.

It seems like this all took place last week because, well, it was last week—seven days that seem like a long, long time ago.

Since then my thoughts have been a blur as my soul does its best to absorb the news. *Should I get a second opinion? But he's the best of the best. Do I get another opinion from someone who is less than the best?*

I have argued with him; I have pitted my other doctors against him; I have asked repeatedly from every conceivable angle. But his answer is the same. *My heart is no longer able to handle the stress of any sort of invasive surgical procedure. I'm officially "inoperable."*

I don't know where we go from here. I'm sorry. There is nothing left for us to do.

Nothing left to do?! Who does this guy think he is? He's the best. Certainly he can come up with something! Maybe he just doesn't understand what this means. I need this surgery. Without this surgery, there will be no further surgeries. I dare him to look me in the eyes and hear me when I tell him what his "no" means: a problem with my cervical spine will go untreated. A number of smaller fatty tumors wrapped around my spine from my neck to my back will go unremoved. And most urgently, my shoulder. My orthopedic surgeon needs to get in

> "Please know that there has been no mistake." They were simple words that didn't quite compute; answers that weren't unexpected, just shocking. After all these years, I should be an expert at this—at getting bad news.

there ASAP. It's ready to rupture and completely shred my tendons at any moment. If this shoulder isn't repaired, it will come apart.

He has pushed the issue with the cardiologist.

I don't know where we go from here . . . .

I tell you what he doesn't know; he apparently doesn't know what this means for my life. Is he going to come over to my house and pick things up for me? Is he going to hug my husband for me? Is he going to wipe away my tears the next time I try to get out of my bed or wheelchair and the throbbing and burning pain shoots through that shoulder? No. He isn't. But that's what I have to look forward to. I wish I could say that I navigated this last week with finesse, but it's been really, really tough. Anger leads me toward the edge of depression as continued pain fuels the despair of a new reality:

There is nothing left for us to do.

This is new territory for me and for those I love. Through dogged determination, hope, and an incurable desire to overcome, we have always found an alternate route—some sort of option, something else to do to keep this old body alive. Our will has always found a way. We've always known that we had a fight on our hands and we have battled through countless medical procedures to keep the breath breathing, the heart thumping, the thoughts coming. I've always had something to do. There's always been some sort of solution to each problem. But not anymore. After going under the knife eleven times, there will be no more surgeries. They don't know what else to do. And I don't know what to do either. Another barrage of thoughts: *Why?! Why?! What now? Load up on the pain meds. Sleep it away. Be careful, very careful with the shoulder...and don't think about it. Why? Why?*

I've been here before, of course, at the crossroads of faith and despair . . . that place where darkness seems impenetrable, where pain clouds everything and the future is so undefined, so vague and so full of fear. Yes, I've been here before, and I know where to go. It's closet time again. Time to let it all out, raise the fist of frustration, release tears of despair, and talk friend-to-friend with the only One who does know. Through the darkness—one more time, until I discover it—one more time:

The defiant candle of hope—a bending, dancing flame that flickers alone—rebelling against the storm of broken expectations, pain and death.

. . . and death. So this is what it comes down to, death, the great equalizer for all humanity. *I'm sorry. There is nothing left for us to do.* Life, it turns out, is terminal after all.

I know; I know I'm not the first one to face this. As Beuchner said, the story of one of us really is the story of all of us. I'm only walking in the footsteps of every soul who has gone before me. I'm only crossing a milestone that brings me consciously closer to that inevitability. I'm in the home-stretch of an amazing journey. A journey that has taken me to the edge of my dreams and beyond— the dream to find true love, denial of my maternal dream to have my own child, and through the ultimate

> "I don't know where we go from here. I'm sorry. There is nothing left for us to do."
> *Nothing left to do?!*
> He's the best. Certainly he can come up with something!

earthy sacrifice of others, the season of disease-free living. Having faced death in the trauma of cardiac arrest, I lived to discover my true identity as a child of God, defying that old mirror.

It's been a good ride. Very few regrets and great memories. Along the way I've believed more in hope than reality. But what I'm finding now is that the focus of my hope is changing—not by choice, but by necessity. This is a new season. It's time to take inventory, time to give thanks, time to say good-bye, time to go for it again with the intent that I can help create a legacy of hope and healing to all who suffer from the chronic, malignant, terminal condition called life. The focus is changing, the clock is ticking and I don't know for sure when the alarm will go off. So I have to ask the question with new, heartfelt gravity:

What if today is all I have?

If today is all I have, I need to be ready for tomorrow. Facing physical mortality can bring great clarity to the soul. I believe that I have three very distinct parts: body, soul, and spirit. As I've been so rudely reminded this week, my body's days are numbered. It's like I'm waiting to exhale—but I know I can't hold my breath forever. One day, one way or the other, my spirit will be released from this beat-up body and enter the timelessness of eternity. If I die, what will happen? No, let me rephrase that: *When* I die, what happens? Will I be able to choose to die? Will it be a conscious letting go of everything and everyone that I've held so dear on this earth, or will death be forced upon me? I've learned to fight so hard, I'm not sure I'm any good at surrender. Will I be willing to wave the white flag when the time comes? Will death come with a jolt, like it did with the cardiac arrest, or will it come as a slow fade as vital organs shut down?

So many questions. The answers will be clear enough in the moment, yet just knowing with new certainty that "the moment" will come is forcing me into a new sense of honesty and even more questions:

- ✧ Am I certain about where I stand with God? Once I breathe my last, there will be no second chances to make things right with Him (Hebrews 9:27).

- ✧ Have I been playing a religious game all these years or have I sincerely placed my trust in Jesus to forgive me? If I admit that I sin, He promises to cleanse me (1 John 1:9).

- ✧ Have I really asked Christ into my life? If I open that door, He says He will come in (Revelation 3:20).

- ✧ Do I believe that I really belong to Jesus and that He is my life? My life was never really mine in the first place (Galatians 2:20).

I don't know that I've ever *not* believed these things. But it sure doesn't hurt to take an inventory of my soul just to make sure—just to make sure that I've got everything ready for the trip—kind of like double-checking to make sure I have my ticket *before* I get to the airport.

When I think that today might be all I have, I must confess that I get very, very sad. I love life. I really, really hate to see it all end. It's been such a good ride. All the things I've done, all that I've learned—it's been so real, so passionate, so . . . fun. But wouldn't it be a waste to get so focused on losing these blessings that I miss the opportunity to say thanks for the gift of all that was?

Of course, it's hardest to lose those things I am most thankful for: Indescribable thankfulness for my mom, my dad, my sister; for the army of friends and professionals who fought the battles beside me. It's unthinkable, actually—the thought that we will

> There's always been some sort of solution to each problem. But not anymore.

be separated. Our souls blend together like the colors of a rainbow glowing in the evening sun. As that sun dips below the horizon, how will we distinguish between the fading colors?

And Greg. Greg. Our souls don't just blend; the pressures of the pain and the power of agape love—have they not forged our hearts into one single beating unit? How, might I ask, can we ever become two again? Do we leave half of our selves with each other, or will both of us die when by death we must part? Each night, falling asleep and facing an uncertain dawn, Greg and I hold hands. Sometimes I wake up at two or three in the morning and we're still holding hands. It's almost as if were holding on for dear life. How in the world will we ever say good-bye?

But if today is all I have, I must learn to say those words. The certainty of my departure demands it. Imminent death is like a message boy on a bike, slipping an urgent warning into my hand:

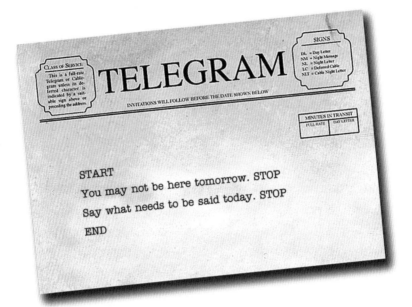

Back in 2000, just prior to my kidney transplant, I took those thoughts to heart. A dark cloud of fear descended on my soul. The reality of my mortality was more present than ever. An obscure concern overwhelmed me; the tentacles of the pink fog seemed to be circling my soul once again. I was certain that the surgery was not going to turn out well. I was worried for my mom; I was worried about leaving Greg; I felt I was abandoning my sister and my dad. I wasn't ready to say "goodbye" to anyone; and yet, just in case my premonition was accurate, I needed to do so.

I locked myself in my room and took out a pen and several sheets of paper. To this day, I don't think I've ever had to experience anything as emotionally difficult as writing those letters of goodbye. But I had no option. I didn't want to leave them without confirming what incredible parents, partners, sisters, friends, and companions they had been. They have made my life beautiful and wonderful—the way that they have tolerated the medical challenges, the way that my dreams disrupted theirs, and I wanted them to know it all. I prayed and wrote for hours that afternoon. Word by word, a sense of calm descended—a sense of closure. *Okay, it's done. I don't have to worry. They'll know.*

And then I wasn't afraid anymore. The fog evaporated and the fear lifted. In fact, I was pretty sure that everything would be okay. I called my minister, Dr. John Dalles and asked if he would come over to see me. He read the letters thoughtfully; we sealed them in envelopes and he took them and locked them in the safe in his office. If the time comes (I mean, *when* the time comes) he will make sure they get them. If nothing else, after decades of banter and jesting with my loved ones, I'm guaranteed to get in the last word.

How much closer are we to the delivering those letters? If I make it through today, we will be one day closer.

Sooooo, *what if today is all I have?* Hmmm. That might be a flawed question, actually. Rather than dwell on hypotheticals, rather than speculate on timing, rather than trying to control the edges of my destiny, shouldn't I rephrase that question as a statement? Because in the scope of time, today *is* all I have. This isn't a "what if." Yesterday is gone; tomorrow *never* comes. The only moment I have is the one I'm standing in right *now*. There is no other possible time to live. I have been given one life and one chance to live it. That chance is *now*.

Paul Tournier once said, "Most people spend their entire lives indefinitely preparing to live." Albert Schweitzer said, "The tragedy of life is what dies inside a man while he lives."[32] I can't stand the thought of that. While I still breathe, while my heart still beats, while thoughts still flicker in my mind, I want to live now, and nothing can stop me from doing so. Every moment is a chance to make a difference, an opportunity to give thanks, an invitation to spread hope, even through the fog of pain. Yes, there is that pain thing again—the price we pay for the deep richness of things that really matter. The pain is getting more intense recently; it threatens to totally consume my consciousness most of the time. But now, standing on a new threshold, I can choose to be thankful not only for the gift of the pain, but the fact that I'm going to be liberated from it relatively soon.

> It's closet time again. Time to let it all out, raise the fist of frustration, release tears of despair, and talk friend-to-friend with the only One who does know.

Disease-free, pain-free living. Not just for a while, but for forever and ever. Wow. I really can't imagine . . . .

When I woke up this morning, the heavy cloud of pain and depression cleared slightly. Though the pain persists, I force the thought, *I want to be worthy of this day. I want to live worthy of the faith that I claim and the prayer that I practice. If there's anything that I can do to glorify God for what He has done for me, that's what I want to do.* If I wake up tomorrow morning not breathing, well so be it.

Today *is* all I have.

Life has amazing potential. Period. We are responsible to pursue this potential no matter what our circumstances. Period. That's not a rah-rah locker room speech to a team that's down by eighty points at half time. This is a real challenge to seize the day with full respect for present pain and difficulties. After Tim Hansel's climbing accident, he went on to create a dynamic outdoor adventure ministry for troubled teens. But he is the first to admit the harshness of his day-to-day experience:

Mine is only a muffled triumph, joy mingled with still ever constant pain and unjustifiable gladness of merely being alive. The daily confrontations often leave me less than the best.

But still something ever new keeps emerging

Hope—now deeper, more enduring
Love—yes, but in unsentimental dailyness
Faith—not enough to move mountains
but just enough to keep me in muffled triumph.[33]

Christopher Reeve and Lance Armstrong found new purpose in their wounds. The injuries and the diseases gave them new reason to live and fight for a better world. My hero, Joni Eareckson Tada, found that her quadriplegia was actually a vehicle that took her places she never could have walked, places big and small where she could share the hope of Christ—the hope that she had come to know *through* her injury. Hansel is right. Ours is a muffled triumph—*but it is a triumph* every time I see that the past is irretrievable, that tomorrow never comes, and that today is all I have.

Comedian Lilly Tomlin once said, "I always wanted to be somebody. Maybe I should have been more specific." Because I still have today I can be ever more specific about the "somebody" I want to be and become. But

> Each breath buys me one more chance to reach out for that defiant candle of hope that bends and dances alone, flickering in the storms of darkness.

that takes focus. I still have the chance to be responsible with by body—to care for it with wisdom and intention. In a world where I am bombarded with thoughts and things that are not important, I still have the chance to refuse the items that aren't at the top of my priority list so I can focus on those I know are most significant. Whether I have ten decades or ten minutes left, realizing that my time is limited should press me toward an immediate urgency to figure out what's important to me and what I'm going to do about it. *And then I can go for it.* I'm very fond of this popular motto:

> Life, it turns out,
> is terminal after all.

Life is not a journey to the grave with the intention of arriving safely in a pretty and well preserved body . . . but rather to skid in broadside, thoroughly used up, totally worn out, and loudly proclaiming "Wow! What a ride!"

~ Author Unknown

I know I've got the "thoroughly used up, totally worn out" part down. I'm a body donor, but what's left to take?! I can see some doctor looking at my cadaver, scratching his head and saying, "Hmmm, that earlobe doesn't look too beat up. Do we have anyone who needs an earlobe transplant?"

And what about *Wow! What a ride?* I think I've got that part down too, at least so far. It's uncharted territory ahead. How will I navigate this next (and probably last) season of life? By embracing today with all I have, moving ahead as best I can, using my will to find the way, and singing a personal prayer that my sister captured for me in a song:

LINDA'S SONG

It seems I've been here a million times, on my knees, Lord I pray.
Asking for the strength I need to get through every day.
Along this journey I've traveled, the road seems long and rough
but there's so much I want to see, that I need your healing touch.

Chorus:
So I ask you, O Lord, to hear my prayers once more.
Give me the Courage to make it through the darkness.
I have seen the greatest of your love and I will never give up.
For the love that surrounds me makes me whole.

I put my trust in you, knowing that I have no control.
But the fear I feel is greater than my body can endure.
I need you now, as always, like footprints in the sand.
To carry me out of this pain and hold my trembling hand.

Chorus:
So I ask you, O Lord, to hear my prayers once more.
Give me the Hope to see the end of my life's darkness.
I have seen the greatest of your love and I will never give up.
For the love that surrounds me makes me whole.

My courage will not fail, though your plan seems so unclear.
I never feel alone. I know your healing hands are here.
I feel I can make it out of the shadow of the unknown
because within me your grace and mercy have grown.

Chorus:
So I ask you, O Lord, to hear my prayers once more.
Show me the Light so I can make it through the darkness.
I have seen the greatest of your love and I will never give up.
For the love that surrounds me makes me whole.

I have learned to embrace each day as I used to seize each of my presents piled under the Christmas tree of my childhood. *This week, more than ever*, I see each day as an undeserved gift from my God, each one waiting to be unwrapped and savored— even when the taste is sweet, bittersweet—or even just very bitter— each breath buys me one more chance to reach out for that defiant candle of hope that bends and dances alone, flickering in the storms of darkness.

> Live each day as if it is your last . . . and one day, you will be right.
>
> ~ Unknown

Yes, I'm *still* happiest when I wake up breathing—*but that might just be because I don't know any better*. The exchange of air through the lungs, the pulsating movement of blood in a vein, the billions of electrical impulses that form a thought in the mind; life is an amazing gift—*and a temporary one*.

Why? Because today is all I have. And that is enough for now.

Through the darkness—
one more time,
until I discover it—
one more time:

*The defiant candle of
hope—a bending,
dancing flame that
flickers alone—rebelling
against the storm of
broken expectations,
pain and death.*

Morning has broken,
    like the first morning . . .

                    ~ Eleanor Farjeon

Epilogue: Morning Has Broken

O N SUNDAY, JANUARY 23RD, 2011, Linda woke up breathing, again.

More than two years had passed since the doctor labeled her "inoperable" for any elective surgery. The months had been a blurred mixture of birthdays and medicine and holidays and accidents and parties and ambulances . . . still she defied all expectations. The last week had been filled with a flurry of drastic life-supporting measures, yet her vitals had stabilized and her "numbers" looked pretty good. That morning, her breathing tube was removed. When her family arrived mid-morning her father, Karl, was greeted with the sweetest words a father could ask for: "Happy Birthday, Daddy." (It was his 75th.)

For the next three hours she talked and laughed. It appeared that she had pulled "the magic rabbit out the medical hat" once again. But by afternoon, Linda had talked herself out of breath

. . . literally. She was weak and worn out and placed back on life support. Over the next two days, as her body gave way one more time, she descended into unconsciousness still determined to hold fast to life—her soul never, ever surrendering.

Her body, however, had reached the inevitable. For decades the family and medical staff had done all they could to sustain it . . . to give her one more day. Now, when the doctor pulled Greg aside to talk about options, he faced the unimaginable: There were no more options.

Two evenings later, the family that had kept her strong for so long surrounded her one last time, keeping a silent, peaceful vigil at her side through a long night. At 7:45 in the morning, January 27th, Linda Nordyke Hambleton took her last breath, exchanging her endearing hope for life on earth for the never-ending hope of Life in eternity!

"At the very moment Linda died," Greg recalls, "the sun came streaming through the window into her room in Florida Hospital's Ginsburg Tower. This seemed supernatural in a sense, since her window faced west. Later, when I went outside and looked up, I realized that the sunlight that came into her room had been reflected off the glass of the new Diabetes Institute across the street. Surely this was a sign of Linda's future impact on the world of diabetes not only at this hospital but everywhere."

The next day, in his church office, Dr. John Dalles took the letters out of his safe and handed them to Linda's family. The words, written with tears nearly a decade before, came alive on the pages again. "If you are reading this . . . I am gone," they read. She went on to tell each of them "thank you" and reminded them to always look up. She assured them that she was infinitely better off and told them to never look back—unless it was with laughter and thanks. In closing, she left her final words to all.

Remember these things:
Life is truly amazing—live it well.
Happiness is always waiting to happen to you—let it.
Peace comes from the knowledge you are not alone . . .
ever. God is with you always.

I am waiting for you . . .

Linda

ACKNOWLEDGEMENTS

*T*O ACKNOWLEDGE THE TEAM OF PEOPLE WHO have kept me alive and make that life worth keeping would take an entire book in and of itself. God knows who you all are. Both He and I thank you so very much. Thank you for enriching and extending my time here on this side of the silver-lined clouds! I am particularly thankful for the following people who have given so much of their own lives so that I can have mine:

My junior prayer warriors, Max and Morgan. An aunt couldn't ask for a more awesome nephew and niece. You are the children I always dreamed of!

Samuel E. (Ned) Crockett, MD. Thank you for giving me two of my three life dreams!

Joseph W. Warren, MD. Thank you for protecting "Jean," my new kidney, and everything she is connected to.

Joel D. Greenberg, MD. Thank you for long hours, long nights and giving so much of your heart to keep mine going!

Florida Hospital Orlando. Thank you all for being a wonderful, safe, and Christ-centered place to spend so much of my time as well as being a true model of the best a hospital can aspire to. Your current and future patients are truly blessed to be in your care.

There are too many of you to name, but a special thanks goes to the patient advocates, physicians, and nurses who so often brought me back from the brink, particularly: Uday K. Ranjit, MD, Madhu Banda, MD, Andrew S. Martin, MD, James J. McClelland, MD, Sigfredo Aldarando, MD, Timothy C. Childers, MD, Rafael A. Cortez, MD, Arnaldo Isa, MD, Tracy Truchelut, MD, Howard B. Finklestein, DPM, and Herbert Mendelsohn, MD.

The EMTs of Casselberry Station 21. Where would I be without you?!

My dear friends Dr. Des Cummings Jr., and his beautiful wife Mary Lou. Thank you for over a decade of prayers, comfort, love, and the opportunity to tell others about you and your amazing hospital and care—but most of all for helping me to tell my story that I might help others in their time of need.

My dear girlfriend Penny "PJ" Jones. Thank you for always making time to visit me every day in the hospital, for giving so much of you—friendship, love, comfort, advice, and "Starbucks coffee visits." You are my Heart Sister!

The nurses and techs that have cared for me over the years. Thank you for your care, comfort, always making sure I am as comfortable as possible, and the prayers you have held up on my behalf—you are angels earthbound!

Frank and Nancy Hambleton, my mother- and father-in-law. You welcomed me into your family and hearts when I married your son and have always made me feel more like your daughter than an in-law. I love you both.

Last, but certainly not least, my precious "BFF" Brenda Ferguson Lange. We have known each other and been a part of each other's lives for more than thirty-six years. You have been a special part of my life and especially my heart. You can make me smile with a hug, a few of your kind words, and a visit when I need it most. You have a special ability to make me feel beautiful even when I'm sure I look my worst! You truly have a gift of amazing friendship! I am so lucky to be on the receiving end of that gift!! I know we will be together as long as I live.

NOTES

1. M. Scott Peck, *The Road Less Traveled* (New York: Simon and Schuster, 1978), 15.

2. See the work of Elisabeth Kubler-Ross, for example, including *On Death and Dying.*

3. Tim Hansel, *You Gotta Keep Dancing* (Colorado Springs: David C. Cook, New Edition, 1998), 15.

4. Lance Armstrong, with Sally Jenkins, *It's Not About the Bike* (Crows Nest, NSW; Australia, 2000), 99.

5. Frederick Buechner, *The Sacred Journey* (San Francisco: Harper and Row, 1982), 46.

6. Hansel, op cit, 68.

7. Ibid, 89.

8. Christopher Reeve, *Nothing is Impossible* (New York: Ballantine, 2004), 30.

9. Hansel, op cit, 31.

10. Philip Yancey, *Disappointment with God* (Grand Rapids: Zondervan, 1988), 17.

11. Ibid, 204.

12. Ibid, 158.

13. Ibid, 165.

14. Ibid, 187.

15. Ibid, 183.

16. Ibid, 157 .

17. Helen Keller, "Three Days to See," (*Atlantic Monthly, 1933. Copyright American foundation for the blind*).

18. As quoted by Tim Hansel, *Holy Sweat*, (Nashville: W Publishing Group, 1987), 130.

19. Randy Pausch, *The Last Lecture* (New York: Hyperion, 2008), 79.

20. Joni Eareckson Tada, *Joni*, (New York: Bantam, 1978), 79-80.

21. Hansel, *Holy Sweat*, 175.

22. Ibid, 144.

23. Ibid, 57.

24. Buechner, op cit, 46.

25. Hansel, *You Gotta Keep Dancing*, 111.

26. Ibid, 53.

27. Ibid, 91.

28. Eugene Kennedy, *The Pain of Being Human* (Garden City, NY: Image Books, 1972), Introduction.

29. Joni, 37

30. Eareckson Tada, op cit, 120-21.

31. Hansel, *You Gotta Keep Dancing*, 79-80.

32. Ibid, 47.

33. Ibid, 137.

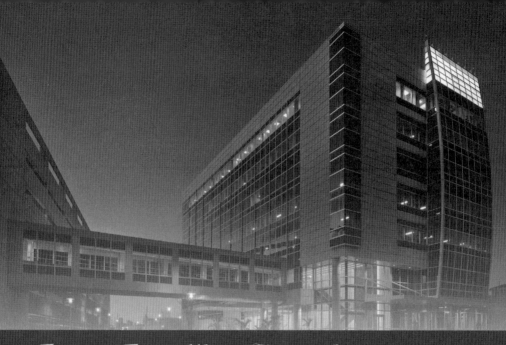

"For us, the Florida Hospital Diabetes Institute meant peace of mind because we knew we could get the help we needed there."

—Bonnie Nordyke (Linda Hambleton's Mother)

How You Can Help

The Florida Hospital Diabetes Institute is one of the nation's most comprehensive diabetes institutes, providing expert clinical care, accredited diabetes education programs, and recognized research protocols. Today the institute provides outstanding services that positively impact tens of thousands of patients.

Florida Hospital established a partnership with Sanford Burnham Medical Research Institute which helped form the Translational Research Institute for Metabolism and Diabetes (TRI). Through the TRI, the Diabetes Institute patients will be among the first in the world to access leading-edge research projects and innovative new treatments focused on diabetes, metabolism, and obesity.

You can honor Linda by supporting her chosen charity, the Florida Hospital Diabetes Institute. A portion of the proceeds from this book will go to the Diabetes Institute.

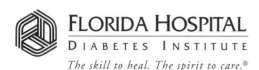

FLORIDA HOSPITAL
D I A B E T E S   I N S T I T U T E
The skill to heal. The spirit to care.®

Florida Hospital Diabetes Institute
2415 North Orange Avenue, Suite 501
Orlando, Florida 32804
(407) 303-2822
www.FloridaHositalDiabetes.com

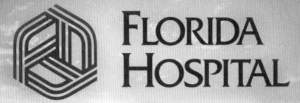

FLORIDA HOSPITAL

The skill to heal. The spirit to care.

Florida Hospital Celebration Health

Florida Hospital Altamonte

GINSBURG

Florida Hospital Winter Park

Florida Hospital Orlando

Florida Hospital East Orlando

Florida Hospital Apopka

Florida Hospital Kissimmee

About Florida Hospital

For over one hundred years the mission of Florida Hospital has been: *To extend the health and healing ministry of Christ.* Opened in 1908, Florida Hospital is comprised of eight hospital campuses housing over 2,200 beds and twenty walk-in medical centers. With over 17,000 employees—including 2,000 doctors and 4,000 nurses—Florida Hospital serves the residents and guests of Orlando, the No. 1 tourist destination in the world. Florida Hospital cares for over one million patients a year. Florida Hospital is a Christian, faith-based hospital that believes in providing Whole Person Care to all patients – mind, body and spirit. Hospital fast facts include:

- **LARGEST ADMITTING HOSPITAL IN AMERICA**. Ranked No. 1 in the nation for inpatient admissions by the *American Hospital Association*.

- **AMERICA'S HEART HOSPITAL**. Ranked No. 1 in the nation for number of heart procedures performed each year, averaging 15,000 cases annually. MSNBC named Florida Hospital "America's Heart Hospital" for being the No. 1 hospital fighting America's No. 1 killer—heart disease.

- **HOSPITAL OF THE FUTURE**. At the turn of the century, the *Wall Street Journal* named Florida Hospital the "Hospital of the Future."

- **ONE OF AMERICA'S BEST HOSPITALS**. Recognized by *U.S. News & World Report* as "One of America's Best Hospitals" for ten years. Clinical specialties recognized have included: Cardiology, Orthopaedics, Neurology & Neurosurgery, Urology, Gynecology, Digestive Disorders, Hormonal Disorders, Kidney Disease, Ear, Nose & Throat and Endocrinology.

- **LEADER IN SENIOR CARE**. Florida Hospital serves the largest number of seniors in America through Medicare with a goal for each patient to experience a "Century of Health" by living to a healthy hundred.

- **TOP BIRTHING CENTER**. *Fit Pregnancy* magazine named Florida Hospital one of the "Top 10 Best Places in the Country to have a Baby". As a result, *The Discovery Health Channel* struck a three-year production deal with Florida Hospital to host a live broadcast called "Birth Day Live." Florida Hospital annually delivers over 8,000 babies.

- **CORPORATE ALLIANCES**. Florida Hospital maintains corporate alliance relationships with a select group of Fortune 500 companies including Disney, Nike, Johnson & Johnson, Philips, AGFA, and Stryker.

- **DISNEY PARTNERSHIP**. Florida Hospital is the Central Florida health & wellness resource of the *Walt Disney World* ® Resort. Florida Hospital also partnered with Disney to build the ground breaking health and wellness facility called Florida Hospital Celebration Health located in Disney's town of Celebration, Florida. Disney and Florida Hospital recently partnered to build a new state-of-the-art Children's Hospital.

- **HOSPITAL OF THE 21ST CENTURY**. Florida Hospital Celebration Health was awarded the *Premier Patient Services Innovator Award* as "The Model for Healthcare Delivery in the 21st Century."

601 East Rollins Street, Orlando, FL 32803 | www.FloridaHospital.org | (407) 303-5600

HEAL*THY*
MIND | BODY | SPIRIT

HEALTHY LIVING RESOURCES

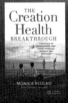

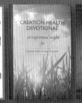
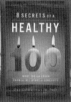
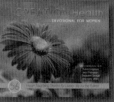

FLORIDAHOSPITALPUBLISHING.COM · HEALTHPRODUCTS@FLHOSP.ORG · (407) 303-1929

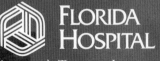

FLORIDA HOSPITAL
AMERICA'S TRUSTED LEADER
FOR HEALTH AND HEALING